The Effect
of Disease States
on Drug
Pharmacokinetics

A Symposium

Sponsored by
Basic Pharmaceutics Section
ACADEMY OF PHARMACEUTICAL SCIENCES

123rd Annual Meeting
AMERICAN PHARMACEUTICAL ASSOCIATION
New Orleans, Louisiana
April, 1976

The Effect
of Disease States
on Drug
Pharmacokinetics

Leslie Z. Benet, *Editor*

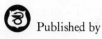 Published by
AMERICAN PHARMACEUTICAL ASSOCIATION
ACADEMY OF PHARMACEUTICAL SCIENCES
2215 Constitution Avenue, N.W.
Washington, DC   20037

International Standard Book Number: 0-917330-11-0
Library of Congress Catalog Card Number: 76-43119

© 1976; All Rights Reserved
AMERICAN PHARMACEUTICAL ASSOCIATION
2215 Constitution Avenue, N.W.
Washington, DC   20037

Printed in the United States of America

CONTENTS

List of Contributors vii

Preface xi

INTRODUCTION

1. New Areas of Research, *William G. Crouthamel* 1

PART I. BODY PERFUSION

2. Pharmacokinetics in Disease States Modifying Body Perfusion,
   Grant R. Wilkinson 13

3. Gastrointestinal Absorption of Drugs in Patients with Cardiac
   Failure, *Leslie Z. Benet, Andreas Greither, and Wolfgang
   Meister* 33

PART II. HEPATIC AND METABOLIC FUNCTION

4. Pharmacokinetics in Disease States Modifying Hepatic and
   Metabolic Function, *Malcolm Rowland, Terrence F. Blaschke,
   Peter J. Meffin, and Roger L. Williams* 53

5. Hepatic Drug Clearance in Chronic Liver Disease, *Robert A.
   Branch and David G. Shand* 77

6. Pharmacokinetic Implications of Chronic Drug Treatment in
   Epilepsy: Carbamazepine, *Rene' H. Levy, William H. Pitlick,
   Allan S. Troupin, and John R. Green* 87

PART III. PROTEIN BINDING

7. Pharmacokinetics in Disease States Changing Protein Binding,
   William J. Jusko 99

8. The Effect of Uremia, Cardiopulmonary Bypass and Bacterial
   Infection on Serum Protein Binding, *William A. Craig, Merle A.
   Evenson, and V. Ramgopal* 125

9. Clinical Implications of Interindividual Differences in
   Plasma Protein Binding of Drugs and Endogenous Substances,
   Gerhard Levy 137

PART IV. RENAL FUNCTION

10. Pharmacokinetics in Disease States Modifying Renal Function, *Peter G. Welling and William A. Craig* 155

11. The Influence of Renal Disease on the Elimination of Procainamide and the Accumulation of N-Acetylprocainamide, An Active Metabolite, *Thomas P. Gibson, Edward Matusik, and William A. Briggs* 189

12. Multiple Dose Pharmacokinetics of Gentamicin in Man: Evaluation of the Jelliffe Nomogram and the Adjustment of Dosage in Patients with Renal Impairment, *Paul A. Michelson, William A. Miller, John F. Warner, Leona W. Ayers, and Harold G. Boxenbaum* 207

Subject Index 247

LEONA W. AYERS, M.D.
Director, Clinical Microbiology
Ohio State University Hospitals
Columbus, Ohio 43210

LESLIE Z. BENET, Ph.D.*
Professor of Pharmacy and
*   Pharmaceutical Chemistry*
School of Pharmacy
University of California,
*   San Francisco*
San Francisco, California 94143

TERRENCE F. BLASCHKE, M.D.
Assistant Professor
Department of Cardiology
School of Medicine
Stanford University
Stanford, California 94305

HAROLD G. BOXENBAUM, Ph.D.*
Senior Scientist
Department of Biochemistry and
*   Drug Metabolism*
Hoffmann-La Roche Inc.
Nutley, New Jersey 07110

ROBERT A. BRANCH, M.R.C.P.*
Assistant Professor of Medicine
*   and Pharmacology*
Department of Pharmacology
Division of Clinical Pharmacology
Vanderbilt University
Nashville, Tennessee 37232

WILLIAM A. BRIGGS, M.D.
Chief, Nephrology Service
Walter Reed Army Medical Center
Washington, D.C. 20012

WILLIAM A. CRAIG, M.D.*
Assistant Professor of Medicine
University of Wisconsin
*   and*
Chief, Infectious Disease
Veterans Administration Hospital
2500 Overlook Terrace
Madison, Wisconsin 53705

WILLIAM G. CROUTHAMEL, Ph.D.*
Associate Professor of
*   Pharmacy*
Department of Pharmacy
School of Pharmacy
University of Maryland
Baltimore, Maryland 21201

MERLE A. EVENSON, Ph.D.
Professor of Medicine
University of Wisconsin
1300 University Avenue
Madison, Wisconsin 53706

THOMAS P. GIBSON, M.D.*
Assistant Chief
Nephrology Service
Walter Reed Army Medical
*   Center*
Washington, D.C. 20012

JOHN R. GREEN, M.D.
Deceased

ANDREAS GREITHER, cand. med.
Berghamerstrasse 7
8206 Bruckmühl
West Germany

*Symposium speaker

WILLIAM J. JUSKO, Ph.D.*
Associate Professor of
    Pharmaceutics
State University of New York
    at Buffalo
            and
Director, Clinical Pharmaco-
    kinetics Laboratory
Millard Fillmore Hospital
3 Gates Circle
Buffalo, New York 14209

GERHARD LEVY, PHARM.D.*
Distinguished Professor of
    Pharmaceutics
Department of Pharmaceutics
School of Pharmacy
State University of New York
    at Buffalo
Buffalo, New York 14214

RENE' H. LEVY, Ph.D.*
Associate Professor of
    Pharmaceutical Sciences
    and Neurological Surgery
School of Pharmacy BG-20
University of Washington
Seattle, Washington 98195

EDWARD J. MATUSIK, B.S.
Research Chemist
Division of Biochemistry
Walter Reed Army Institute
    of Research
Washington, D.C. 20012

PETER J. MEFFIN, Ph.D.
Assistant Professor
Department of Cardiology
School of Medicine
Stanford University
Stanford, California 94305

WOLFGANG MEISTER, M.D.
Clinical Pharmacology Fellow
Division of Clinical Pharmacology
Department of Medicine
School of Medicine
University of California,
    San Francisco
San Francisco, California 94143

PAUL A. MICHELSON, M.S.
Assistant Clinical Professor
    of Pharmacy
College of Pharmacy and Allied
    Health Professions
St. John's University
Jamaica, New York 11432

WILLIAM A. MILLER, PHARM.D.
Director, Division of
    Clinical Pharmacy
College of Pharmacy
University of Tennessee
Memphis, Tennessee 38163

WILLIAM H. PITLICK, Ph.D.
Assistant Professor of
    Biopharmaceutics
School of Pharmacy
University of Pittsburgh
Pittsburgh, Pennsylvania 15261

VADAKEPAT RAMGOPAL, M.D.
Fellow, Infectious Diseases
Department of Medicine
University of Wisconsin
Madison, Wisconsin 53706

MALCOLM ROWLAND, Ph.D.*
Professor of Pharmacy
Department of Pharmacy
University of Manchester
Manchester M13 9PL
England

DAVID G. SHAND, M.R.C.P.,Ph.D.
Associate Professor of
    Medicine and Pharmacology
Department of Pharmacology
Division of Clinical
    Pharmacology
Vanderbilt University
Nashville, Tennessee 37232

ALLAN S. TROUPIN, M.D.
Assistant Professor
Neurological Surgery
Director, Seizure Clinic
    RC-76
University of Washington
Seattle, Washington 98195

JOHN F. WARNER, M.D.
*Division of Infectious
    Diseases
Department of Medicine
Ohio State University
    Hospitals
Columbus, Ohio 43210*

PETER G. WELLING, Ph.D.*
*Associate Professor of
    Pharmaceutics
School of Pharmacy
University of Wisconsin
Madison, Wisconsin 53706*

GRANT R. WILKINSON, Ph.D.*
*Associate Professor of
    Pharmacology
Department of Pharmacology
Vanderbilt University
Nashville, Tennessee 37232*

ROGER L. WILLIAMS, M.D.
*Clinical Pharmacology Fellow
Division of Clinical Pharmacology
Department of Medicine
School of Medicine
University of California,
    San Francisco
San Francisco, California 94143*

PREFACE

Pharmacokinetics has been defined as the study of the time course of absorption, distribution, metabolism, and excretion of drugs and their corresponding pharmacologic, therapeutic, or toxic response in animals and man. It is usually stated that the development of mathematical models are virtually essential to the interpretation of the kinetic phenomena. Before 1970 the majority of research work in pharmacokinetics was concentrated on those drugs which could be analyzed easily using simple (and often imprecise and nonspecific) spectrophotometric and microbiological techniques. In this pre-1970 stage, a great deal of effort was directed toward the development of sophisticated mathematical models which, at times, were much more complex than was needed to describe the limited data available. Initiates to the field often indicated that they believed that the mathematical modeling techniques had far outstripped the meager amount of good data describing the time course of drugs or metabolites measured using a specific assay.

During the past six years the analytical capabilities for measuring drug and metabolite levels have improved considerably. More and more drug studies are being reported in which specific analytical techniques have been developed so that drug concentrations may be measured accurately at levels seen during normal drug dosing. Surprisingly, as our analytical techniques began to improve, we found that the sophisticated mathematical models previously developed were not adequate. It became increasingly difficult to delineate which of the many pharmacokinetic parameters should be utilized in comparing drug absorption and disposition in normal subjects with pharmacologic response data. This uncertainty became particularly acute when investigators began to study drug kinetics in the patient as opposed to the healthy volunteer. Only in the last three years have pharmacokineticists begun to look at their data in terms of pharmacokinetic parameters which more closely approximate physiologic processes, i.e., the introduction of clearance concepts and the delineation of the differences between blood-flow limiting processes and organ-clearing capacity processes. Approximately one-half of the chapters in this book discuss disposition processes in terms of the intrinsic clearance of the organ, a term which was generally unknown in the field of pharmacokinetics two years ago.

With the emergence of these new mathematical approaches to analyzing pharmacokinetic data, we felt that a symposium directed to the examination of the effect of disease states on pharmacokinetics would be well timed. Only a relatively few papers have appeared in the literature on this subject and the participants in this symposium are among the leaders in the design and execution of such studies. Previously, in April 1972 the Pharmacology and Toxicology section of the APhA Academy of Pharmaceutical Sciences organized a symposium on Pharmacokinetics in the Disease State. Many of the speakers at that symposium also are contributors in the present work. Although the proceedings of the 1972 symposium were not published, those of us who attended the meeting gained very useful insights even though much of the material descriptively presented at that time could not be organized into a useful format utilizing the pharmacokinetic techniques then available. The papers from the present 1976 symposium also contain a great deal of descriptive information, however these papers also contain the ideas and methodology upon which changes of drug kinetics in disease states may be evaluated and predicted. Today, in contrast to the 1960's, mathematical model development lags behind the analytical techniques and it is probable that new methods of data analysis and comparison will develop within the next few years using the basic concepts presented in this book.

The timeliness of a symposium in 1976 on the effect of disease states on pharmacokinetics was suggested by Dr. William G. Crouthamel who served as the symposium chairman and presented the introductory paper. This symposium was not organized with respect to particular disease states or particular drug classes, but with reference to "physiologic" functions which may be modified by the disease state and thus affect the absorption and disposition processes of the drugs administered to patients to alleviate the particular disease. The four basic areas chosen for discussion were: I. Changes in blood flow; II. Changes in hepatic and metabolic function; III. Changes in protein binding; and IV. Changes in renal function. Each section was organized with a lead speaker who concentrated on presenting a general overview of the disease states which could modify a particular "physiologic" function and who then described the latest pharmaco-kinetic modeling techniques which were being utilized in evaluating these changes and their effects on drug kinetics. These lead speakers were selected not only because they were carrying out studies in a particular area but also because they had been instrumental in the development of the modeling techniques which are now receiving wide-spread attention in the analysis of kinetic data. The second and third speakers in each section described the active research programs being carried out in their laboratories which serve to delineate the effect of disease states on drug kinetics. Of course, none of the above "physiologic" processes can be isolated as having a unique effect on drug kinetics. Obviously, changes in blood flow will change hepatic and renal elimination processes, protein binding changes may signifi-cantly effect distribution and elimination processes, and a disease state in one organ group may cause changes in another set of organs, i.e., the hepato-renal syndrome. However, after reviewing pre-symposium manuscripts and abstracts, attempts were made to assign specific areas to specific speakers to avoid redundancy. Every effort was made to edit chapters so the reader could readily see how one particular chapter was coordinated with others in the book and could easily find all aspects of a particular topic of interest.

This book begins with a general orientation to the effect of disease states on pharmacokinetics and with some specific comments on the use of animal models as preliminary tools in elucidating potential kinetic changes. Chapter 2 presents an overview of pharma-cokinetics in disease states which may modify blood flow. Clearance concepts are introduced and described with particular emphasis on how changes in flow may be differentiated from changes in the intrinsic

clearance. A particular disease state, congestive heart failure, which
markedly modifies body perfusion, and how these changes can and do affect
the absorption process is discussed in Chapter 3. An overview of drug
kinetics in patients with hepatic dysfunction is presented in Chapter 4.
Particular emphasis is given to the intrinsic clearance concept. The
effect of changes in protein binding on the kinetics of metabolism are
discussed. The effect of chronic liver disease on hepatic clearance is
examined in Chapter 5. The authors attempt to delineate how drugs may
be used as diagnostic agents in evaluating the severity of liver disease
and in predicting kinetics of other drugs having metabolic patterns
similar to the marker. The kinetics of a particular drug, carbamazepine,
in a particular disease state, epilepsy, are discussed in Chapter 6.
Chapter 7 presents a comprehensive review of changes in drug-binding
components and of factors which alter drug-protein binding. Specific
discussions of changes in the binding of phenytoin, corticosteroids,
and digoxin are elucidated. The authors of Chapter 8 review how uremia
and bacterial infection as well as a surgical procedure, cardiopulmonary
bypass, may alter serum protein binding as opposed to that found in
normals. The clinical implications of interindividual differences
of plasma protein binding specifically for warfarin, phenytoin, and
bilirubin are discussed in Chapter 9. Up to the present time, the most
progress in evaluating the effects of disease states on drug kinetics has
been made in the area of altered renal function. Chapter 10 presents a
comprehensive review of the field and presents a compilation in tabular
form which may be used in adjusting drug dosage for those compounds
which are particularly influenced by changes in renal function. Chapter
11 describes the effect of renal disease on a particular antiarrhythmic
agent, procainamide, and especially emphasizes the importance of recognizing the effects of renal disease on the accumulation of the active metabolite of this compound. A discussion of the applicability of various
dialyzers in the elimination of this drug from anephric patients is also
presented. The effect of changes in renal function on gentamicin kinetics
is discussed in Chapter 12. While the title of this chapter is directed
toward a particular dosage adjustment scheme, the authors review all of
the methodologies employed with gentamicin and suggest the differences
from study to study more probably reflect differences in gentamicin
standards used, than in a variation in the effects of renal disease on
drug elimination. The index was prepared with particular emphasis on
including references to all of the drugs and disease states mentioned
within the twelve chapters. Uniform terminology and symbols were used
throughout the book.

    In a field where developments are occurring so quickly it is critical
that the publication of the proceedings of a symposium should occur soon
after the oral presentations. I am indebted to the authors for their
help in allowing us to prepare a completed version of the proceedings of
the symposium within three months of its presentation. I am especially
grateful to all those involved since an added burden was put upon them
because the editor was on sabbatical during the period when the symposium was organized and presented, and when the papers were edited and
typed in final form. I thank Dr. William Crouthamel for serving as the
symposium chairman, and I thank Dr. Sidney Riegelman and Dr. Crouthamel
for serving as the moderators during the symposium. I am very

appreciative of the assistance that Ms. Linda McLaughlin and Dr. William F. McGhan of the Academy office gave to me. I am pleased that we were able to publish this book before Bill McGhan retired as Executive Secretary. The organization and efficiency which he has lent to all Academy proceedings will be missed. I also wish to thank Professor Luzius Dettli for providing me with excellent facilities, patience, and good counsel, which allowed me to carry out much of the work involved in putting together this volume while in Basel, Switzerland. Finally, I gratefully acknowledge the invaluable help which my administrative assistant, Ms. Linda Kiefer, and my secretary, Ms. Naomi Sinai, have given to me during the planning, preparation, and final assembling of this text.

San Francisco, California   Leslie Z. Benet
July 21, 1976

INTRODUCTION

Chapter 1

NEW AREAS OF RESEARCH

William G. Crouthamel

A Symposium entitled "Clinical Pharmacokinetics" was held at the 17th
National Meeting of the American Pharmaceutical Association Academy of
Pharmaceutical Sciences in New Orleans on November 13, 1974. At this Symposium the general concepts of clinical pharmacokinetics were discussed,
and the proceedings published (1). This present Symposium is a natural out-
growth of the previous one held approximately 1½ years ago and represents both
the evolution of new knowledge and the growing realization that the disease
under treatment and its severity can dramatically influence the optimum
dosage regimens of many drugs. The reasons for the evolution are varied, but
undoubtedly were greatly influenced by recent developments in the disciplines
of analytical chemistry, clinical pharmacology and therapeutics. Based on
more sensitive assays for both parent drug and active metabolites, it is now
possible to better define therapeutic concentration ranges of drugs and thus
more accurately determine when drug concentrations are within the desired
range. In the past, many effects probably due to diseases were masked by
problems in assay sensitivity, intrasubject variation, patient non-compliance
and interaction with other drugs concomitantly being administered to the
patient. While these problems continue at the present time, there is a greater awareness of how these factors can influence drug therapy and help explain
some of the sources of variation. The number of clinical pharmacokinetics
laboratories presently in operation or in developmental stages is growing.
This has served a dual purpose - to increase the data base for drugs under
study and to increase the awareness of the role of pharmacokinetics in drug
therapy. As a result of these factors there has been increased interest in
the effects of disease states on drug pharmacokinetics. Since the importance
of clinical pharmacokinetics is to individualize drug therapy, an appreciation
of the patients disease states and the effects which these disease may have
on drug therapy is important.

From an historical perspective the spectrum of disease has dramatically
changed in the last 50 years. Tuberculosis, which ranked second as a cause
of death in 1900 does not appear in the 10 most frequent fatal disease in 1965
(2). As public health has improved in the United States, many once fatal diseases have been greatly reduced in importance and more people are living
longer lives. Instead of dying from typhoid fever or pneumonia, people are
surviving to acquire the chronic illnesses of advanced age - cardiovascular
disease, diabetes and cancer. The aged population (65 years and over) has
almost doubled between 1930 and 1974, while the population under 14 has declined during the same period. This is reflected in the three leading causes
of death at the present time - heart disease, cancer and stroke - with heart

1

disease being responsible for more deaths than cancer and stroke combined. These statistics suggest that in the future we should expect to see more of the diseases related to the aging process. The average person in 1974 suffered 17 days of restricted activity, 7 days of bed disability, lost 5 days of work due to illness, and averaged 5 physician visits. In addition, 28% of the population suffered an accident during this period, and the average person spent 8% of their income on direct health care services (3). These figures point out the profound impact of disease on our society, even in a nation of relatively good health.

Diseases are, by definition, processes which alter the normal functions of the body, and these alterations lead to the manifestations of the disease. Since the body handles many drugs and endogenous substances similarly, it is not surprising that diseases which alter the pharmacodynamics of endogenous substances also alter the pharmacodynamics of drugs. For example, renal insufficiency produces an accumulation of endogenous substances as well as drugs normally excreted by this route. Similarly, diseases which impair the liver's ability to metabolize and excrete endogenous substances can also have the same effect on drugs, although this process is much more difficult to define than in the case of the kidney. Congestive heart failure and other pathologic conditions compromising cardiac function can reduce blood perfusion of the tissues of absorption, distribution and elimination and can profoundly alter the time course and disposition of a number of drugs. Also, since only the free (or unbound) drug is usually available to interact with receptors and thus elicit a pharmacological response, changes in the protein binding of drugs would be expected to change the availability of drug to the receptor as well as to other organs of the body. These topics will be discussed in much more detail in the 11 chapters which follow.

Even some of the peripheral components of diseases may have in themselves a significant effect on drug pharmacokinetics, although the relationship may be difficult to determine. For example, seriously ill patients are usually confined to bed whereas less seriously ill patients are usually ambulatory. Detailed physiological studies have shown significant differences in body function during sleep and recumbency but the effects of these factors on drug pharmacokinetics have not been carefully evaluated. DiSanto and Wagner (4) studied the urinary excretion of leucomethylene blue and concluded that they could not correlate the diurnal (day-night) variation in urinary excretion of leucomethylene blue with either changes in urinary pH or with urinary flow rate. Tetracycline (5) and erythromycin stearate also appear to have significant day-night effects. Routine pharmacokinetic studies usually require that the volunteers remain "ambulatory and awake." However, drugs are often administered under conditions other than these. Another peripheral component of disease states which can potentially alter drug pharmacokinetics is the general state of the patient. In long term diseases and in the aged, debilitative changes often take place. Since most drugs distribute and bind to some extent in extravascular tissue compartments, deterioration of the body muscle mass and subsequent changes in the fat/lean ratio may result in significant changes in drug pharmacokinetics. Future studies in this area are especially important in view of the advancing age of the general population.

Because most of the data reported in this symposium results from studies conducted in human subjects, I would like to briefly emphasize another approach which can be helpful in understanding the effects of disease states on drug pharmacokinetics. Most disease states are complex entities, hence it is often difficult to properly assign observed pharmacokinetic changes to specific components of the disease. This is particularly true in light of the difficulties encountered in obtaining sufficient blood, urine and tissue samples from ill patients to completely characterize a drug pharmacokinetic profile. An alternate but complementary method to testing drugs in humans is to induce specific components of the disease under study in otherwise healthy animals, thereby allowing an evaluation of only the specific parameters of interest. It is well documented that differences exist between man and animals and between animal species (6), but much useful information can still be gained from this approach.

An example of the above approach is our study of the effects of congestive heart failure, where decreased cardiac output results in decreased blood perfusion of many parts of the body, including the gastrointestinal tract. Because the rate and extent of drug absorption are important determinants of the time course of drug action, we felt it important to delineate the effects which congestive heart failure can have on these parameters. To study this we acutely implanted an electromagnetic blood flow sensor on the mesenteric artery of anesthetized healthy dogs. Intestinal drug absorption was measured at four different times in situ as intestinal blood flow was reduced from normal flow to no flow by occlusion of the artery. Our studies (7) showed that intestinal drug absorption rate decreased as we reduced the rate of intestinal blood perfusion. In comparing these results with quinidine data in congestive heart failure patients, we observed (8) that peak quinidine concentrations occur approximately two hours later in congestive heart failure patients than in normal individuals, and that the estimated rate of drug absorption in the congestive heart failure patients was only one-third of that in normal subjects. In addition, the amount of quinidine absorbed appeared to have been reduced in congestive heart failure, although this could not be definitely determined from this data. Surprisingly, there was no change in the elimination rate constant of quinidine in the congestive heart failure patients as compared to normal subjects, but a large change was found in the calculated volume of distribution. Following intramuscular injection of quinidine, absorption was also considerably slower in congestive heart failure patients and the volume of distribution was reduced. Although long term effects of congestive heart failure on the gastrointestinal tract, including mucosal changes, infarction, and hypoxia, may also alter drug absorption, intestinal perfusion must be considered an important determinant of drug absorption in this disease. A more detailed description of drug pharmacokinetics in congestive heart failure is contained in Chapters 2 and 3.

Elevated serum lipid levels are an endogenous disease of Western man. Plasma lipid levels in American adults are much higher than in many other parts of the world, and this is probably a major reason for the 20th Century epidemic of atherosclerosis and coronary heart disease. Reasons for the high serum lipids in a given individual may be genetic, environmental, or the result of a pathological condition. Hyperlipidemia may involve elevated serum cholesterol, triglycerides, free fatty acids or a combination of these lipids. This areas has received only very recent attention as to the effects which elevated serum lipids can play in drug pharmacokinetics, and is another area in which studies utilizing animal models of specific aspects of the disease appear to be suitable. In man, elevated cholesterol and triglyceride levels lead to varying degrees of atherosclerosis and cardiovascular disease,

3

and result in changes in cardiovascular function and body perfusion. In addition, large elevations in serum lipids are often associated with other pathological conditions such as diabetes. The combination of all these factors makes it difficult to separately evaluate the effects of each on drug pharmacokinetics.

Elevated free fatty acid concentrations are found in a number of clinical conditions including diabetes, infection, hypothyroidism, stress, and reduced caloric intake (9). Thus the observation of a change in the pharmacokinetics of a highly bound drug in the presence of elevated free fatty acid concentrations would appear to have widespread significance. To study the effect of free fatty acid concentrations on drug pharmacokinetics, free fatty acid concentrations were elevated in the rat by direct intravenous infusion of free fatty acids or by the infusion of a free fatty acid precursor (9). The hypolipidemic drug clofibrate was chosen for study because it is a drug of choice in patients with elevated serum lipid levels, and could be expected to be used in the presence of elevated free fatty acid levels. The results of

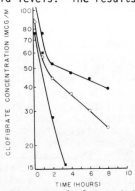

Fig. 1 - Plasma clofibrate concentration as a function of time under control conditions (●) (n=7), elevated free fatty acid concentrations due to infusion of triglyceride emulsion (O) (n=4), or elevated free fatty acid concentration due to direct infusion of linoleate (■) (n=2). The solid line represents the best computer fit. (Reproduced with the permission of the publisher).

the study are shown in Fig. 1. We found that the presence of elevated free fatty acid concentrations decreased the half-life of clofribrate from approximately 19.3 hr in controls to 7.3 hr in the treated animals, and increased the apparent volume of distribution from 0.15 L/kg to 0.20 L/kg. Both clofibrate and free fatty acids are extensively protein bound, and free fatty acids have been reported to displace clofibate from albumin binding sites in vitro (10). Although the importance of this interaction in man cannot be evaluated from this data alone, the pharmacokinetics and protein binding of clofibrate in the rat and man are quite similar (9).

Further studies (11, 12) of the hypotriglyceridemic effect of clofibrate in the rat indicate that the primary effect of this drug is a depression of the hepatic synthesis of triglyceride rather than an alteration of the kinetics of triglyceride turnover. Thus as drug treatment continues and serum lipid levels decrease, a change in the protein binding and the pharmacokinetics of the drug should take place. This may help explain the observation that treatment failures with clofibrate are more prevalent in patients with high initial serum lipid levels than in patients with lower initial lipid levels, although more studies in man are needed to substantiate this relationship. Interestingly, in the rat and probably man, there appears to be two different types of triglyceride synthesized, each with its own half-life. Clofibrate reduces only one of these types so that the "apparent" half-life of triglyce-

4

ride becomes prolonged following clofibrate treatment (11, 12). Thus the relationship between concentrations of triglyceride, free fatty acids and clofibrate is probably a complex one. A more detailed description of the interaction between free fatty acids and drugs binding to albumin in man will be covered in Chapters 7 and 8.

Another potentially important area in which little work has been done is that of drug binding to serum components other than albumin. It is well known that endogenous substances such as lipid soluble vitamins and steroid hormones are transported throughout the body bound to lipoproteins, and studies of drug plasma protein binding have often found discrepancies between the amount of drug bound in plasma and that which could be accounted for by binding to albumin alone. Recent studies have suggested that circulating lipids can influence the action of lipophilic drugs by acting as an additional storage and/or binding depot. The consequences of this, as with binding to albumin, could be a change in the plasma concentration of free drug and quantitative alterations in drug response. The possibility that circulating lipid levels could influence the response of lipophilic drugs is of practical importance in view of the widespread hyperlipidemia encountered in Western man.

To investigate the effect of elevated serum cholesterol concentrations on drug pharmacokinetics, hypercholesterolemia was induced in rabbits by feeding a high cholesterol diet. We found that the hypotensive effect of prostaglandin E_1 and the hypertensive effect of phenylephrine _in vivo_ were significantly decreased in the presence of hyperlipidemia (13). Typical data is shown in Fig. 2. Atherosclerotic related changes in arterial

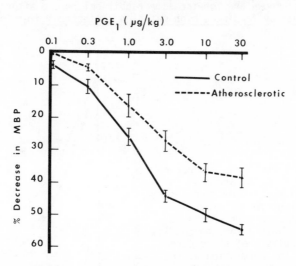

Fig. 2 - Decrease in mean blood pressure in control (n=7) and atherosclerotic rabbits (n=7) produced by prostaglandin E_1. Data represented as mean ± S.E. (Reproduced with the permission of the publisher).

smooth muscle were initially considered as an explanation for the decreased drug response. However, this explanation appeared unlikely since aortic strips from normal and severely atherosclerotic rabbits responded identically to the contractile effects of these drugs in vitro. Addition of a lipid emulsion to the in vitro tissue bath caused a shift in the dose response curve to the right in proportion to the amount of lipid added, and was in general agreement with our in vivo observations. Pharmacokinetic studies of two sulfonamides performed in rabbits before and after induction of hyperlipidemia showed that the primary change in pharmacokinetics was a decrease in the apparent volume of distribution in the presence of hypercholesterolemia. Typical data is shown in Fig. 3 and Table I. In additional studies hyperlipidemic rats which had not yet become atherosclerotic were less responsive

Table I Sulfamerazine Pharmacokinetics in the Normolipidemic
and Hyperlipidemic Rabbit

Condition[a] of Rabbit	Volume of Distribution $V.$ (L)	Rate Constants (hr^{-1})		
		k_{12}	k_{21}	k_{el}
Normolipidemic	1.80	0.487	0.164	1.53
Hyperlipidemic	1.43	0.412	0.233	1.22

[a]The data shown are for the same rabbit before and after induction of hyperlipidemia by feeding a high fat-high cholesterol diet for 6 weeks.

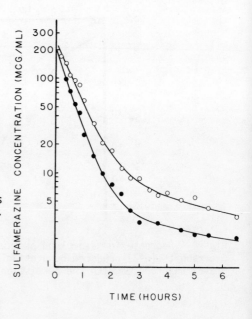

Fig. 3 - Disappearance of sulfamerazine (100 mg/kg I.V.) from the serum of the rabbit before (close circles) and after (open circles) induction of hyperlipidemia by feeding a high cholesterol diet. See Table I for the results of the kinetic analysis of these curves. (Reproduced with the permission of the publisher).

6

to the CNS convulsant effect of the lipophilic drug flurothyl. Thus it appears that hypercholesterolemia can alter the pharmacokinetics of lipophilic drugs presumably by acting as an additional storage or binding site for the free drug. Additional evidence for this hypothesis was found when hypercholesterolemic serum from rabbits administered a sulfonamide was separated into high lipid and low lipid serum fractions by ultracentrifugation. Analysis of these fractions indicated that the sulfonamide concentration in the high lipid fraction was 2-3 times that in the low lipid fraction. Since hypercholesterolemia can fluctuate greatly in disease states altering lipid metabolism, and increases with age, this appears to be an important area for future research in man.

This work as well as the studies with free fatty acids points out the importance of measuring free rather than total drug concentrations. In both cases the primary change which occurs is essentially an alteration in the bound to free drug ratio, and measurement of only total serum drug concentration may result in misleading information. In the studies involving hypercholesterolemia, increased total blood drug concentrations were associated with decreased pharmacological effect; measurement of only total drug concentrations would have been difficult to interpret.

Considerable information is presently available on the pharmacokinetics of drugs such as digoxin, propranolol, lidocaine, the anticonvulsants, theophylline and many of the antibiotics. However, the effects of disease states on even these drugs is not completely understood and much work remains to be done. Drugs are routinely tested for efficacy in diseased patients, but most pharmacokinetic studies are performed in healthy adult male volunteers. Thus the pharmacokinetics we usually deal with are "idealized" pharmacokinetics in that the studies were carried out in healthy individuals rather than in the diseased patients whom are the recipients of most medication. In addition, many diseases are multifaceted and consist of a number of sequelae, so that the final resulting pharmacokinetic profile will be the sum total of the various positive and negative effects. An example of such a disease is diabetes, where serum lipids (cholesterol, triglyceride and free fatty acids) are often elevated, metabolism is altered, changes in membrane permeability may occur, and changes in the fat/lean body weight ratio are common. In complex disease states such as this there will probably not be any single parameter which can be uniquely used to correlate with drug pharmacokinetics. In cases such as this the importance of input from a clinical pharmacokinetics laboratory must be emphasized.

Summary

Recent advances in analytical methodology have provided the opportunity to more carefully study the pharmacokinetics of a large number of drugs. With these advances have come an explosion of studies performed in normal human subjects, but little information has appeared on the effects which disease states may have on drug pharmacokinetics. Disease states by definition change the normal functions of the body, so it is not surprising that drugs administered under these conditions could have altered pharmacokinetics. Because most disease states are complex entities, it is often difficult to properly assign observed pharmacokinetic changes to specific modalities of the disease. Animal models incorporating specific components of the disease under study can provide information on the relative contribution of each of the individual components of the disease. This approach has been used to study the potential effects of congestive heart failure and hyperlipidemia on drug pharmacokinetics. In dogs, decreased intestinal blood perfusion resulted in decreased intestinal drug absorption rate, and correlated with observed quinidine pharmacokinetic changes in human congestive heart failure patients. In the rat model, elevated free fatty acid concentrations altered clofibrate pharmacokinetics by competing for plasma albumin binding sites. In the rabbit model, elevated serum cholesterol concentrations resulted in altered drug pharmacokinetics and in vivo activity due to increased drug binding in plasma. Since these conditions are present in a large number of disease states, they need to be more carefully evaluated in human subjects.

Acknowledgements

The serum lipid studies were conducted in collaboration with Richard J. Cenedella, Ph.D., Department of Pharmacology, West Virginia University Medical Center, Morgantown, West Virginia. These studies were supported in part by grants from Merck Institute for Therapeutic Research, The West Virginia Heart Association, and the West Virginia University Computer Center.

References

1. G. Levy (ed.) Clinical Pharmacokinetics - A symposium, American Pharmaceutical Association Academy of Pharmaceutical Sciences, Washington, D.C., 1974.

2. L.E. Burton and H.H. Smith, Public Health and Community Medicine, Williams and Wilkins, Baltimore, M.D., 1970, pp. 145.

3. Source Book of Health Insurance Data 1975-76, Health Insurance Institute, New York, N.Y., 1975, pp. 64.

4. A.R. DiSanto and J.G. Wagner. Pharmacokinetics of highly ionized drugs II. Methylene blue absorption, metabolism and excretion in man and dog after oral administration. J. Pharm. Sci. 61: 1086-1090 (1972).

5. W.H. Barr, J. Adir, L. Garrettson. Decrease of tetracycline absorption in man by sodium bicarbonate. Clin. Pharmacol. Ther. 12: 779-84 (1971).

6. W.G. Crouthamel, C.R. Abolin, J. Hsieh, J.K. Lim. Intestinal pH as a factor in selection of animal models for bioavailability testing. J. Pharm. Sci. 64: 1726-7 (1975).

7. W.G. Crouthamel, L. Diamond, L.W. Dittert, J.T. Doluisio. Drug Absorption VII: Influence of mesenteric blood flow on intestinal drug absorption in dogs. J. Pharm. Sci. 64: 664-671 (1975).

8. W.G. Crouthamel. The effect of congestive heart failure on quinidine pharmacokinetics. Am. Heart J. 90: 335-339 (1975).

9. W.G. Crouthamel and R.J. Cenedella. Clofibrate pharmacokinetics: Effect of elevation of plasma free fatty acids. Pharmacology 13: 465-473 (1975).

10. A.A. Spector, E.C. Santos, J.D. Ashbrook, J.E. Flectcher. Influence of free fatty acid concentration on drug binding to plasma albumin. Ann. N.Y. Acad. Sci. 226: 247-258 (1973).

11. R.J. Cenedella, W.G. Crouthamel, H.F. Mengoli. Intestinal versus hepatic contribution to circulating triglyceride levels. Lipids 9: 35-42 (1974).

12. R.J. Cenedella and W.G. Crouthamel. Halofenate and clofibrate: Mechanism of hypotriglyceridemic action in the rat. J. Lipid Res. in press (1976).

13. R.J. Cenedella, W.G. Crouthamel, G.C. Bierkamper, D.P. Westfall, Alteration of drug pharmacodynamics by hyperlipidemia. Arch. Int. Pharmacodyn. Ther. 218:229-311 (1975).

I. BODY PERFUSION

Chapter 2

PHARMACOKINETICS IN DISEASE STATES

MODIFYING BODY PERFUSION

Grant R. Wilkinson

Classical pharmacokinetics has developed elegant and sophisticated mathematical techniques for the analysis of drug amount and/or concentration/time
data, and this has proven valuable in a variety of applications concerning
drug action and usage. The main emphasis has been upon use of descriptive
models (1-3), and, although a few of the derived parameters may have direct
physiological reality, eg, blood clearance, the majority of these terms have
no immediate association with the involved in vivo processes. There has,
therefore, been a tendency to overlook the fact that the experimental data is
the end result of the interaction of a number of controlling biological processes. Recognition of these limitations has led, in recent years, to the
development of more physiologically oriented models of drug disposition,
which permit identification of the role and importance of certain of the in
vivo processes. In view of the transportational function of the blood, it is
not surprising that hemodynamic considerations are of major significance in
this type of approach. All of the processes involved in drug disposition,
namely, absorption, distribution and elimination, may be influenced by perfusion considerations. Whereas the principles and concepts involved are
reasonably simple, their validation and quantitative significance have been
primarily limited to the processes of absorption and hepatic elimination.

Alterations in organ perfusion may arise because of either changes in
the magnitude and/or the regional distribution of the cardiac output, and
may involve physiological, pathological, surgical or drug related events.
Generally, these causative factors also result in perturbations in other
determinants of drug disposition which may exaggerate or dampen any effects
produced by the changes in blood flow. It is,therefore, quite difficult to
quantitatively define the precise contribution of any perfusion changes, and
this is particularly so in man. As a result,the clinical role and importance
of changes in perfusion is frequently inferential, based upon animal experiments designed to demonstrate the validity of certain principles or to investigate a model of the disease state.

Drug Absorption and Hemodynamics

The role of organ perfusion, especially pulmonary blood flow, in the uptake and distribution of general anesthetics is well recognized (4). Increased perfusion of the lungs by increasing cardiac output leads to enhanced
uptake of the anesthetic into the systemic circulation, whereas lowering the

13

output has the opposite effect; the changes being most pronounced with those gases exhibiting the greatest blood solubility. This has particular implications for the use of these agents in patients suffering from shock where the reduced output if combined with increased ventilation may lead to unexpected levels of highly soluble anesthetics, sufficient to fatally depress the already compromised circulation. The use in such patients of less soluble agents, such as cyclopropane and nitrous oxide, carries less risk of this type of untoward effect. Since the pharmacological action of the anesthetic agent may include depression of the cardiac output it is also possible for the anesthetic to affect its own uptake and disposition, although the clinical significance of this is questionable (4).

Similar principles to those involved in the pulmonary uptake of gases apply to the absorption of drugs at other sites in the body, ie, drugs with high membrane permeabilities, such as very lipid soluble or pore-diffusible substances, exhibit perfusion-limited absorption, whereas the absorption rates of drugs possessing low permeabilities are independent of blood flow. The absorption of several compounds after intramuscular injection has been investigated with respect to the blood supply to the different sites of injection. Insulin absorption has been found to correlate with regional blood flow (5),and deltoid injection of lidocaine gave higher peak plasma levels than lateral thigh injection,which in turn gave higher concentrations than gluteal injection (6,7). This corresponds to the rank order of the blood flow to each muscle group (8). Similar differences in plasma levels was observed with diazepam after injection into the thigh and buttocks (9), and exercise of the thigh increased the level after injection into this site (10).

The influence of blood supply on the in vivo oral absorption of drugs is more difficult to evaluate. Animal studies have indicated that altered intestinal blood flow can significantly alter the rate and extent of absorption dependent upon the drug's absorption characteristics (11). This has been suggested to explain, in part, differences in plasma level/time curves after oral administration in normal subjects and patients exhibiting cardiovascular abnormalities. For example, procainamide (12) and hydrochlorthiazide (13) in cardiac failure,and aprindine (14) and disopyramide (15) in acute myocardial infarction. Details of other studies in both man and animals are described in Chapters 1 and 3.

Drug Clearance and Hemodynamics

The limitations of an elimination half-life or rate constant in providing information on the functional ability of an organ(s) involved in drug elimination is now well recognized, although many otherwise competent investigators still persist in linking these terms with a specified elimination process(es). It is clear that drug clearance, either of a single organ or the sum of all the eliminating organs, is a far better measure of the efficiency of irreversible drug removal from the circulation. In addition, the use of the clearance of drug which is not bound to any of the components of the circulating blood (free drug clearance, CL_u) overcomes many of the problems associated with alterations in drug binding. More importantly, free drug clearance is an indication of the removal of the presumed pharmacologically active drug moiety. Several recent articles have reviewed these and

14

other aspects of the clearance concept (16-18).

Perhaps, not sufficiently recognized is the importance of drug clearance being estimated with respect to the drug within the blood, rather than plasma, if physiological interpretations are to be made of the estimate. This is because drug is delivered to the clearing organ by the blood, which, from a mass transfer standpoint, usually behaves as a single compartment; drugs equilibrate sufficiently rapidly between the erythrocytes and the plasma so that any drug in the red blood cells is available for clearance (19). Ideally, then, blood concentrations should be determined. There are, however, several practical problems and inconveniences attendant to this approach; hence, it is not unusual to measure the plasma level and to convert this value to the corresponding blood concentration by means of a blood/plasma concentration ratio. Care should be taken, however, to establish that this ratio is a true estimate of drug distribution in the blood delivered to the clearing organ. Recent studies have indicated that artifacts may arise in this ratio as a consequence of the technique used for blood collection, in particular the type of container utilized. Thus, spuriously high blood/ plasma ratios were observed for propranolol (20) and meperidine (21) when one brand of a commercially available type of blood collection tube was used relative to an all-glass system. It was demonstrated that the responsible factor was the stopper of the tube which presumably contains a substance(s) which may be leached out by the blood, and then acts as a displacing agent for the plasma binding of the drugs. A similar phenomenon may also occur with the material of indwelling cannulae which are frequently used in blood sampling (20). The effects of such an artifact is to underestimate the blood clearance derived from plasma concentrations, and errors as large as two-fold have been observed (20). It is also possible that the blood/plasma ratio may be dependent on the site of the blood sampling since the ratio for oxyphenbutazone in the dog (22) was significantly lower in arterial blood (0.91) than in peripheral venous blood (1.08).

The clearance concept is well established in physiology, and investigators in this area were amongst the first to recognize that clearance involved not only the ability of an organ to remove a substrate, ie, the extraction ratio (E), but also the rate at which it was delivered to the organ by the blood (Q), Eq. 1a. Thus, the clearance of chromic phosphate colloid (23-25) and bromosulfophthalein (25,26) in the isolated perfused rat liver was found to be a function of perfusate flow rate. The degree of hepatic arterialization significantly affected the elimination in the dog of hydrocortisone (27) and its hepatic clearance in the sheep was a function of the liver blood flow (28). A relationship was also found between hepatic blood flow and the hepatic removal rate of oxyphenbutazone in the dog (29). Some of these studies also noted that changes in hepatic perfusion led to varying alterations in the efficiency of organ uptake; the extraction ratio decreasing as a consequence of increased flow. This observation makes intuitive sense if the liver is regarded as a reactor; the slower the perfusion rate, the longer the time of contact between the blood and tissue, and there is more opportunity for the reaction to reach completion ie, E→1. Using this approach, Brauer and colleagues (23-26) formulated a model of hepatic clearance in which the relationship between blood flow and extraction was of the form of a cumulative exponential, with the exponent involving a constant and the reciprocal of flow (Eq. 1b). More recently, Levy and Nagashima (30,31) and

Winkler et al. (32) have developed relationships of the same form, the only difference being the functional significance placed upon the constant in the exponent. In contrast to this approach is the model first described by Rowland et al. (16) which is frequently called the perfusion-limited model, Eq. 1c. A basic assumption of this model is that the unbound drug concentration in the emergent blood in the hepatic vein is in equilibrium with the unbound drug concentration in the tissue. In addition, the removal process is conceptualized in terms of the maximal ability of the organ to clear a drug in the absence of any flow-limitations, ie, Q is very high. This has been termed the intrinsic clearance of *total* drug which may be conceptualized in terms of the clearance of drug from liver water (CL_{int}) and the fraction of unbound drug in the blood (f), ie, total intrinsic clearance = $f.CL_{int}$. It is apparent that total intrinsic clearance is equivalent to the constant (K) in the exponent of the exponential model.

$$\text{Clearance} = Q\ E \qquad\qquad (\text{Eq. 1a})$$

$$\text{Exponential Model} = Q\left[1 - e^{-\frac{K}{Q}} \right] \qquad\qquad (\text{Eq. 1b})$$

$$\text{Perfusion-limited Model} = Q\left[\frac{f.CL_{int}}{Q + f.CL_{int}} \right] \qquad\qquad (\text{Eq. 1c})$$

Although the two models provide a superficially similar functional relationship between blood flow, drug extraction and clearance there are differences as indicated in Fig. 1. The divergency is greater at low flow rates where the exponential model predicts a relative better extraction and larger clearance than the perfusion-limited approach. Both Brauer et al. (24, 25) and Whitsett et al. (29) noted that the experimentally observed extraction ratios of radiocolloid and oxyphenbutazone, respectively, were lower than that predicted from the exponential model. In the isolated perfused rat liver the elimination of dl-propranolol at varying doses was consistent with the perfusion-limited model (33). The effects of altering perfusate flow on the acute and steady-state concentrations of dl-propranolol, lidocaine and phenytoin after intravenous and intraportal injection also fitted the predictions of this model better than the exponential one (34). A similar conclusion has been drawn by Pang and Rowland based on their studies with lidocaine in the perfused rat liver (35). Consequently, the presently available experimental evidence is most supportive of the perfusion-limited model for describing the inter-relationship between blood flow to an eliminating organ such as the liver and the functional ability of the organ as assessed by either clearance or extraction.

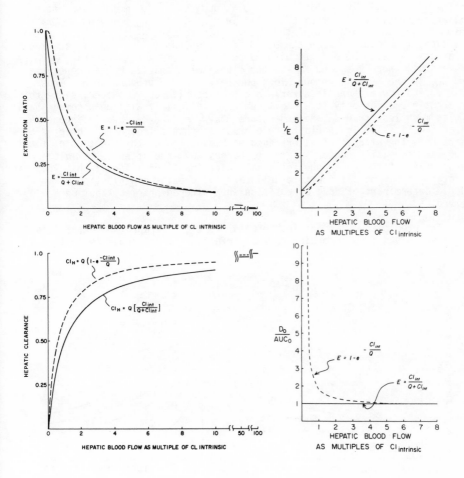

Fig. 1. Comparison of the predicted relationships between organ blood flow and clearance, extraction ratio, its reciprocal, and the ratio D_0/AUC_0 according to the exponential and perfusion-limited models of drug elimination (Eq. 1a-c, and where $Cl_{intrinsic}$ (Cl_{int}) is equivalent to $f.CL_{int}$).

Hepatic Clearance

The perfusion-limited model describing drug clearance involves two physiological variables, namely, the hepatic blood flow (Q) and the hepatic total intrinsic clearance. The latter is a measure of the inherent overall ability of the liver to irreversibly remove *total* drug by either metabolism and/or biliary excretion. If required, total intrinsic clearance may be separated into components indicative of the free intrinsic clearance (CL_{int}), and the fraction of unbound drug in the blood (f) (see Chapter 4). Intrinsic free clearance may also be defined with respect to enzyme kinetics; $CL_{int} = V_{max}/(K_m + C_{HV})$, where V_{max} and K_m are the classical Michaelis Menten constants and C_{HV} is the hepatic venous blood concentration of unbound drug. Thus, dose dependency of hepatic clearance can be considered. However, since this apparently applies only to a small number of drugs, it will be assumed that C_{HV} is much less than K_m and, therefore, $CL_{int} = V_{max}/K_m$, and is independent of dose. Finally, it should be re-emphasized that although this chapter concerns only the effects of alterations of blood flow on the kinetics of total drug, the causative factors of these changes may, and often do, simultaneously affect the other physiological determinants of disposition. Thus, in practice it may be difficult to delineate the precise contribution of any single determinant of drug disposition when altered pharmacokinetics are observed.

The predicted relationships between hepatic clearance and extraction, and liver blood flow according to the perfusion-limited model is indicated in Fig. 2.

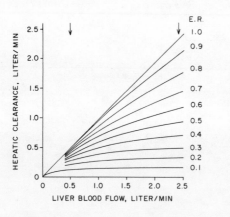 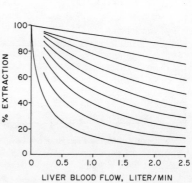

Fig. 2. Relationships between liver blood flow and hepatic clearance, and extraction ratio for drugs with varying total intrinsic clearances. The individual curves reflect a 10% stepwise change in extraction at a normal flow of 1.5 liter/min, and the arrows indicate the normal physiological range of flow in man (18). (Reproduced with permission of the publisher).

18

Dependent on the value of the drug's total intrinsic clearance relative to flow, a family of curves are obtained when the latter parameter is altered. For a drug with a high total intrinsic clearance, decreasing flow leads to a relatively small but inversely proportional change in the extraction ratio. If total intrinsic clearance is small, a larger increase in extraction occurs as flow decreases. Accordingly, the effects of changes in flow on hepatic clearance are somewhat compensated by an opposing trend in extraction for drugs with small total intrinsic clearances and the hepatic clearance is virtually independent of flow. If, however, total intrinsic clearance and extraction are high, then hepatic clearance is essentially a reflection of the delivery rate of the drug to the liver, and changes in blood flow will produce almost proportional changes in clearance. For drugs with intermediate total intrinsic clearances, hepatic clearance is partly flow dependent. Since the elimination half-life and the area under the blood concentration/time curve after intravenous administration (AUC_{iv}) are both inversely proportional to the hepatic clearance, changes in hepatic blood flow also cause alterations in these parameters (Fig. 3). Thus, for a low clearance drug, half-life and AUC_{iv} are independent of alterations in hepatic flow while the opposite applies to a drug with a high intrinsic clearance and extraction ratio. The magnitude of the change will be dependent upon the relative importance of hepatic clearance in the total elimination of the drug.

A slightly more complex situation applies when the drug is administered orally under different conditions of hepatic blood flow. This is because the drug is subject to first-pass or presystemic elimination in the liver prior to reaching the systemic circulation. Since the fraction of the absorbed dose which escapes this phenomenon must be equal to (1-E), it is clear that alterations in flow will affect the drug's bioavailability (Fig. 2); an increase in flow resulting in an increased bioavailability and vice-versa. On the other hand, once the drug is in the systemic circulation, clearance by the liver will be affected by flow according to the perfusion-limited model described above. Thus, the clearance and elimination half-life may be altered dependent upon the total intrinsic clearance of the drug. Importantly, the change in bioavailability (1-E) is exactly offset by the change in hepatic clearance. Therefore, although the shape of the blood concentration/time curve after oral administration may be affected by changes in hepatic blood flow, the area under this curve is flow independent (Fig. 3). In fact, for a drug totally eliminated by the liver, the ratio of the absorbed oral dose to the area (AUC_0) is the total intrinsic clearance of the drug (18,34,36). The apparent paradox, wherein AUC_0, or its equivalent average steady-state blood level, is flow-independent while after intravenous administration AUC_{iv} is flow dependent, has a corollary. Namely, for a drug which is eliminated only by hepatic clearance AUC_0 is equal to the AUC of the hepatic venous concentration after systemic administration of that dose of drug which reaches the liver after oral administration. These predictions have recently been confirmed for propranolol, lidocaine and phenytoin in the perfused rat liver both in the acute and steady-state situation (34) and, as mentioned previously, these findings provide strong support for the validity of the assumptions of the perfusion-limited model. This study also indicated the practical possibility of determining total hepatic blood flow in the absence of portacaval shunting without recourse to catheterization of the hepatic vein. This is possible because for a fully orally absorbed drug which is eliminated solely by the liver, $Q = D/(AUC_{iv}-AUC_0)$ (18). In two normal male volunteers the hepatic blood flow estimated by this technique was 1.6 and 1.8 liters/min, and similar good agreement with published values has also been obtained in the monkey and anesthetized rat (unpublished observations). Unfortunately, Gram and colleagues used plasma rather than blood concentrations in their investigations of this approach with imipramine and nortriptyline in man (37,38).

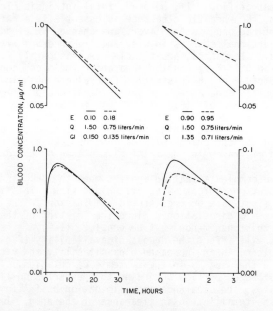

Fig. 3. Effects of decreasing liver blood flow on the blood concentration/time curves after intravenous (upper panels) and oral administration (lower panels) of equal doses of two drugs which are totally metabolized by the liver. The left panels refer to a drug with a total intrinsic clearance equivalent to an extraction ratio of 0.1 when blood flow equals 1.5 liter/min , and the right panels to a drug with a total intrinsic clearance equivalent to an extraction ratio of 0.9 (18). (Reproduced with permission of the publisher).

The above theoretical considerations provide the basis for examining the effects of perturbations in hepatic blood flow on drug clearance and removal caused by altered cardiac output and/or redistribution of the blood. Factors modifying both of these values have recently been reviewed (17) and some of the more pertinent stimuli are indicated in Table I. Only those related to disease will be further considered.

Table I. Some Factors Which Alter Hepatic Blood Flow

	Increased Flow	Decreased flow
Physiological	Supine posture Food intake, digestion	Upright posture Thermal stress Exercise Volume depletion
Pathological		Congestive heart failure Cirrhosis Circulatory collapse Renovascular hypertension
Pharmacological	Glucagon Isoproterenol Phenobarbital	Propranolol Norepinephrine Dimethylbiguanide Anesthetics

Pathological Variations: A number of different disease states are known to alter the hepatic blood flow (39,40) but there is only limited data on the effects of this upon hepatic drug clearance. A pathological decrease in cardiac output appears to produce vasoconstriction of the splanchnic circulation and the fall in liver blood flow is usually proportional or slightly greater than the reduction in output. Congestive heart failure produces a decrease in the plasma clearance of lidocaine in man (41,42). In such patients the cardiac index was generally decreased leading to a proportional change in hepatic blood flow (43). Significantly, the steady-state blood concentration was inversely proportional to the estimated liver blood flow (43,44). It has also been suggested that the clearance of the demethylated metabolite of lidocaine may also be reduced in congestive heart failure (44). A similar phenomenon has been observed for aldosterone (45). Since these compounds normally have hepatic extraction ratios such that flow-dependency would be predicted, it is highly probably that the altered drug delivery rate is an important factor in these situations. However, it is not possible to rule out the involvement of other factors affecting drug clearance.Certainly in the hemorrhaged monkey changes in total intrinsic clearance probably occur in addition to altered liver blood flow, since there is a larger change in the clearance of lidocaine from the blood than would be predicted from the 30% reduction in cardiac output (46). Shock of varying etiology also affects the half-life of indocyanine green, a drug whose hepatic clearance in normal man is blood flow-limited; in 131 critically ill patients with shock this value was prolonged two to six-fold (47). It would follow that the clearance of other high total intrinsic clearance drugs would be similarly affected. A logical extension of this would be the use of a flow-dependent marker drug to predict the clearance and, therefore, steady-state levels, of another flow-dependent drug. This approach has recently been investigated using the clearance of indocyanine green, which can easily be determined within a few minutes, to predict the rate of infusion of lidocaine necessary to provide steady-state antiarrhythmic blood levels several hours after initiating therapy (48).

In liver disease there are alterations not only in the functional ability of the hepatic cells but also in hepatic circulation. Varying degrees of abnormality of portal and total liver blood flow occur dependent upon the nature and severity of the disease. In individuals with cirrhosis the estimated total flow is significantly reduced (49,50). However, in viral hepatitis flow has been found to be essentially normal (51) or to increase as much as 30% over control values or those measured after clinical recovery (52,53). In addition, there is also the possibility of extra- and intra-hepatic anastomoses which shunt blood away from functional cells. Such abnormalities may be quite significant; in alcoholic liver disease, up to 62% of mesenteric and 80% of splenic flow may undergo hepatic shunting (54), and from 4 to 66% of portal blood entering the liver may not pertuse the parenchyma because of intrahepatic shunts (55). Thus, it is not surprising that the clearances of drugs with apparently high total intrinsic clearances in normal individuals are reduced in patients with liver disease. This has been reported for lidocaine (41,42), propranolol (56, Chapter 5) and indo-cyanine green (50,57-59, Chapter 5). An intriguing finding is that the reduction in clearance of these types of compounds apparently parallels that of drugs with low total intrinsic clearances (Chapter 5). This would imply that, at least in chronic liver disease,functional, in contrast to total, hepatic blood flow may be related in some fashion with free intrinsic clearance. Further investigation into this possibility is obviously required. Another relatively unexplored area concerning hemodynamics and liver disease is that of the predicted increase in drug bioavailability after oral administration resulting from portacaval anastomoses. This could produce a significant alteration in systemic drug concentrations which would be compounded by the decreased clearance of the drug. Recent animal (60) and human (61) studies have demonstrated the possible magnitude of such changes. In addition, the increased incidence of central nervous system side effects of the schistosomicide, niridazole, in the hepatosplenic form of bilharziasis compared to the intestinal form of this disease has been suggested to be due to this shunting of portal blood away from the liver leading to a reduction in the magnitude of the first-pass effect (62).

Splanchnic blood flow has been reported to be significantly decreased in patients with hypertension, particularly those with renal artery stenosis (63). This appears to be due to redistribution of the cardiac output but the change, although significant, is quite modest (15%). Several pathological conditions, some common (myocardial infarction) others more rare (beriberi) are known to either increase or decrease the cardiac output quite significantly (39,40). Whether these changes have any effects on the clearance of drugs which have flow dependent characteristics of hepatic removal, and which are used in patients with these diseases remains to be investigated. It would also be interesting to know in diseases affecting hepatic blood flow whether the response of the splanchnic circulation to normal physiological stimuli such as posture, stress, food and exercise is in any way altered.

Hemodynamic drug interactions: In so far as drugs are generally administered to cure or alleviate symptoms of disease, consideration of the likelihood of drugs affecting hepatic function by means of a perfusion mechanism would appear pertinent. In addition, study of these hemodynamic interactions have provided much of the experimental evidence for the role and importance of the flow parameter in drug elimination, since reasonably well controlled studies can be designed and performed.

Several drugs have been shown to either increase or decrease liver blood flow and thus affect the hepatic removal of other drugs having a high intrinsic clearance. dl-Propranolol has been used quite extensively in this regard since the l-isomer acutely decreases cardiac output by about 25% and liver blood flow by some 35% in the monkey (64,65). Administration of dl-propranolol to the dog produced a 50% increase in the half-life of lidocaine which could be accounted for by a reduction in hepatic drug clearance secondary to the hemodynamic changes (66). Importantly, the pharmacologically inactive d-isomer caused no change in the disposition of lidocaine. A similar observation, but of lesser magnitude, was made with oxyphenbutazone (22) and this is consistent with the lower total intrinsic clearance of this drug relative to lidocaine. An interesting situation also occurs with racemic propranolol because of its own high total intrinsic clearance and the different activities of its isomers. As a consequence, the pharmacological action of the drug affects its own clearance. Thus, the in vivo clearance of dl-propranolol in the monkey was 25% less than that of the d-isomer, although the calculated total intrinsic clearances were identical (64). Also, in the isolated perfused rat liver, the clearances of the two isomers were equivalent when the perfusate flow was held constant (33). This hemodynamic phenomenon may explain the shorter half-life of d-propranolol compared to dl- or l-propranolol in man (67), although stereospecific hepatic and/or extrahepatic metabolism cannot be entirely ruled out.

Alpha adrenergic agents cause a decrease in hepatic blood flow by constriction of the splanchnic vasculature (68). Accordingly, an affect on the hepatic clearance of highly extracted drugs would be expected. Experimentally, norepinephrine has been shown to decrease the clearance of lidocaine in the rhesus monkey, presumably by this mechanism (46). Of importance in this regard is the fact that these types of vasoactive drugs are often administered in situations where the hepatic blood flow may already be compromised, such as during shock or circulatory collapse.

Anesthesia is also known to decrease the perfusion of the liver along with other hemodynamic changes (69,70). In man, splanchnic vascular resistance increases, probably as a result of the consequences of artificial respiration (71), but in addition the anesthetic agents themselves can alter hepatic blood flow. Cyclopropane decreases liver flow by 33% (72); halothane causes a similar decrease but much more hypotension is present (71); and methoxyflurane causes a much larger decrease in splanchnic blood flow than

23

either of these agents (73). Hypotension produced by spinal anesthesia can result in a reduced hepatic blood supply with the effects being more marked the higher the level of the block (69). There is little evidence in man that morphine, thiopental, pentobarbital or nitrous oxide have any effects on splanchnic blood flow other than the response produced by hypercarbia. Evidence to the effects of these hemodynamic changes on the hepatic clearance of drugs is largely unknown. However, the finding that the clearance of hydrocortisone in the sheep is reduced by more than 50% during pentobarbital anesthesia (28) indicates that this type of interaction occurs and may be quite significant.

It is also possible for pharmacologic agents to increase the liver blood flow thus enhancing the hepatic clearance of flow dependent drugs. Thus, isoproterenol increases the clearance of lidocaine by 40% (46) and glucagon the clearance of propranolol by 14% (74) in the monkey. The shorter half-life in man of the anticoagulant phenprocoumon when dimethylbiguanide is concomitantly administered has also been rationalized on the basis of increased hepatic clearance secondary to blood flow changes (75). Phenobarbital, in the rat and monkey, also increases the liver blood flow (76-78) in addition to its effects on liver mass and enzyme activity. Accordingly, this altered flow may play a role in the well known inductive effect of this drug. However, the relative contributions of altered flow and total intrinsic clearance will depend upon the specific drug, particularly its total intrinsic clearance. Thus, 43% of the increase in d-propranolol clearance after phenobarbital pretreatment of the monkey, initial E=0.56, could be attributed to an increase in total intrinsic clearance; the remaining and major change resulted from an increase in hepatic blood flow (78). On the other hand, increased hepatic blood flow played a minor role (15%) in the increased clearance of antipyrine, since its initial extraction was only about 25% (78). More recent studies with indocyanine green in the rat (79) reinforce this principle and further illustrate the need to carefully differentiate the underlying mechanisms involved in any observed change in drug clearance. Due to a saturable hepatic uptake process, the kinetics of indocyanine green elimination are dose dependent over the dose range 1 to 50 mg/kg, but over the time period studied may be described by a first-order process. Therefore, the results may be regarded as being analogous to the administration of various drugs with different total intrinsic clearances. Phenobarbital pretreatment, but not 3-methylcholanthrene or 3,4-benzpyrene, altered the half-life and blood clearance of the dye from 40 to 48%. Changes in both hepatic flow and total intrinsic clearance were present and the 33% flow increase accounted for 47.8%, 19.2% and 3.3% of the increased clearance at the 1,10 and 50 mg/kg dose levels (Table II). Significantly, when the absolute increase in total intrinsic clearance was expressed per unit weight of liver there was no change compared to the saline control. This would indicate that phenobarbital pretreatment did not produce induction of any protein involved in the hepatic uptake and storage of the dye, and the increase in clearance was due to the presence of a larger normal liver with a proportionally elevated blood flow. The exact contributions of each of these factors are dependent upon the dose of indocyanine green, flow being less important as the dose is increased since this situation reduces total intrinsic clearance. Therefore, proper interpretation of the interaction of drugs with phenobarbital requires knowledge of the initial total intrinsic clearance and the magnitude of any blood flow or total intrinsic clearance changes.

Table II. Changes in Hepatic Clearance, Extraction Ratio and Total Intrinsic Clearance in Saline and Phenobarbital Pretreated Rats, and the Calculated Contributions of Liver Blood Flow and Total Intrinsic Clearance to the Changes in Clearance of Indocyanine Green.

Dose mg/kg		$t_{\frac{1}{2}}$ min.	Blood Clearance ml/min/ 100g, bw (E)	Hepatic intrinsic clearance, ml/min 100g, bw	g/liver	% Increase in Clearance due to	
						Flow	Intrinsic Clearance
1	Saline	2.39	3.07(0.46)	5.68	1.60	47.8	52.2
	Phenobarb.	1.86	4.30(0.48)	8.36	1.59		
10	Saline	4.03	1.21(0.18)	1.48	0.42	19.2	80.8
	Phenobarb.	2.68	1.78(0.20)	2.23	0.44		
50	Saline	29.75	0.19(0.03)	0.196	0.055	3.3	96.7
	Phenobarb.	19.02	0.27(0.03)	0.279	0.055		

Extra-hepatic Clearance

The principles and concepts described with respect to hepatic drug clearance presumably apply to any other organ of elimination. Unfortunately, little or no experimental evidence is available with the exception of the kidney. In this case, despite receiving a similar fraction of the cardiac ouput as the liver, the renal blood flow and glomerular filtration rate are less variable because of autoregulation than is the hepatic blood flow. There is sufficient evidence to suggest, however, that changes in drug delivery rate can affect renal excretion and this is more significant for those drugs which have a high clearance than those which are simply cleared by glomerular filtration. Thus, the clearance of PAH is significantly increased by phenobarbital pretreatment which raises the renal plasma flow by 69% whereas inulin clearance is unaffected (80). Likewise, the renal excretion of phenobarbital is increased by dopamine (81) which as indicated earlier significantly elevates the cardiac output and renal perfusion. Clinical experience also indicates that the renal clearance of many drugs is reduced when renal perfusion is impaired, and modification, usually intuitive, of the dosage regimen is routinely made.

Hemodynamics and Drug Distrubution

Systemic drug clearance is possibly the most clinically important pharmacokinetic characteristic of a drug's disposition, since this parameter controls the average steady-state blood concentration. However, knowledge of
the quantitative fashion in which the drug distributes within the body is of
considerable significance when considering single doses and the elimination
half-life. Altered hemodynamics can apparently affect both the magnitude
and the rate at which distribution equilibrium is attained. The distribution of lidocaine is perhaps the classical example of this type of phenomenon. Patients with congestive heart failure have almost double the plasma
concentration of lidocaine than normal subjects receiving the same intravenous dose, and this is associated with reductions in the initial distribution space and volume of distribution at steady-state (41,42). It was suggested that these findings resulted from the decreased cardiac output and
organ perfusion. Interestingly, the relative decrease in distribution was
approximately equal to the decrease in systemic clearance (vide infra) hence,
there was little overall effect of altered perfusion on the elimination
half-life. Subsequently, the effects of altered perfusion were investigated
in the monkey using hemorrhage to affect cardiac output and blood distribution (46). Based upon blood concentrations, 30% hemorrhage led to a 38%
and 19% decrease in the initial and steady-state volume of distribution,
respectively, and the time to reach distribution equilibrium was prolonged.
These findings were in relatively good agreement with the predictions based
upon a perfusion-limited model of distribution and elimination (82). Additional simulations for the monkey and man predicted that the hemodynamic
effects of hemorrhage and norepinephrine would cause a decrease in the estimated volumes of distribution, while isoproterenol would produce an increase
in these parameters (46). Perfusion changes have also been suggested to
explain the apparent change in distribution of procainamide (12),quinidine
(83) and digoxin (unreported observations) in patients with cardiac failure.
The decrease in cardiac output with age has also been considered to be a
potential factor in the higher plasma levels of morphine which are seen in
older patients immediately after intravenous injection (84).

Altered drug distribution due to an interaction with another drug
possessing cardiovascular activity and, therefore, the potential to change
hemodynamics, has not been specifically studied, but there is data to suggest that this would occur. Thus, the distribution of oxotremorine is dose-
dependent but this is not observed if the profound hypotension caused by its
peripheral cholinergic effect is suitably blocked (85). In a similar fashion the cardiovascular effects of halothane have been predicted to alter its
uptake and distribution (4).

A decrease in the initial volume of distribution of a drug, which is
seen after rapid intravenous administration, and the decrease in the rate at
which distribution equilibrium is achieved in the presence of altered perfusion may be rationalized in terms of a reduced uptake by the involved
organs. However, it is more difficult to explain the differences which are
observed in drug distribution after tissue equilibrium has apparently been
achieved; drug delivery rate would only be expected to affect the rate at
which equilibrium is achieved but not the final state. The changes in lidocaine distribution caused by hemorrhage probably involves an alteration in

the hematocrit since the estimates were based on blood determinations (46). On the other hand, anemia is not a characteristic of heart failure in man but distribution changes apparently occur. Whether these are a result of changes in plasma and/or tissue binding of the drug or the limitations of the kinetic analysis of blood data is not clear (46).

Perspectives

Despite the truism that drugs are used predominantly in diseased patients, it is only relatively recently that there has been more general recognition that the disease-state may have profound effects upon drug disposition, even if a major eliminating organ such as the kidney is not directly involved. Clearer understanding of any pharmacokinetic differences between patients and normal subjects must be based upon a quantitative understanding of the role and importance of the physiological determinants of the disposition processes. Organ blood flow is one of these factors, and it may contribute to a minor or major degree in any of the processes of absorption, distribution and elimination, dependent upon the drug in question. Unfortunately, there are many practical and ethical problems associated with recognizing and defining the magnitude of any changes, particularly in an individual patient. Animal models are of value in demonstrating the validity of a principle or the existence of a specific phenomenon but are of limited value in extrapolating to man. Consequently, only generalizations can be made with respect to the clinical significance of any perfusion based pharmacokinetic changes, and again it must be appreciated that these do not usually occur in isolation from alterations in the other determinants of drug disposition. It is also important to recognize that the normal homeostatic mechanisms limit the magnitude of any perfusion changes. Thus liver blood flow rarely varies more than fourfold and, even for a drug with a high total intrinsic clearance, this in itself will only result in steady-state blood levels from 50 to 200% of those achieved with normal blood flow. As a result, this type of change will only be clinically significant for those drugs which in addition have a low therapeutic index. Similar considerations apply to situations involving altered systemic absorption or distribution. The types of patients most likely to manifest pronounced hemodynamic changes are clearly those with heart failure, shock and/or drug or surgically induced circulatory abnormalities. In these situations, drugs which normally exhibit an important flow dependent disposition process should be administered with prudence. Hopefully, future investigations will permit more definitive therapeutic guidelines for the involved agents.

References

1. M. Gibaldi and D. Perrier. Pharmacokinetics. Dekker, New York, N.Y., 1975.
2. A. Rescigno and G. Segre. Drug and Tracer Kinetics, Blaisdell, Waltham, Mass., 1966.
3. J. G. Wagner. Fundamentals of Clinical Pharmacokinetics, Drug Intelligence Publications, Hamilton, Ill., 1975.
4. E. I. Eger II. Anesthetic Uptake and Action, William and Wilkins, Baltimore, Md., 1974.

5. C. Binder. Absorption of injected insulin. Thesis, Hvidore Hospital
    and Novo Research Institute. 1969, Ejnar Munksgaards Forlag.
6. L.S. Cohen, J.E. Rosenthan, D.W. Horner, Jr., J.M. Atkins, O.A. Matthews
    and S.J. Sarnoff. Plasma levels of lidocaine after intramuscular admin-
    istration. Amer. J.Cardiol. 29: 520-523 (1972).
7. M.L. Schwartz, M.B. Meyer, B.G. Covino, R.M. Narange, V. Sethi, A.J.
    Schwartz and P. Kamp. Antiarrhythmic effectiveness of intramuscular
    lidocaine; influence of different injection sites. J. Clin. Pharmacol.
    14: 77-83 (1974).
8. E.F. Evans, J.D. Proctor, M.J. Fratkin, J. Velandia and A.J. Wasserman.
    Blood flow in muscle groups and drug absorption. Clin. Pharmacol. Therap.
    17: 44-47 (1975).
9. K. Korttila and M. Linnoila. Absorption and sedative effects of diazepam
    after oral administration and intramuscular administration into the
    vastus lateralis muscle and the deltoid muscle. Br. J. Anesth. 47: 857-
    862 (1975).
10. R.A.E. Assaf, J.W. Dundee and J.A.S. Gamble. Factors influencing plasma
    diazepam levels following a single administration. Brit. J. Clin.
    Pharmacol. 1: 343-344 (1974).
11. L. Ther and D. Winne. Drug absorption, Ann. Rev. Pharmacol. 11: 57-70
    (1971).
12. J. Koch-Weser. Pharmacokinetics of procainamide in man. Ann. N.Y. Acad.
    Sci. 179: 370-382 (1971).
13. K.V. Anderson, H.R. Brettell and J.K. Aikawa. C^{14}-Labelled hydrochlor-
    thiazide in human beings. Arch. Int. Med. 107: 168-174 (1961).
14. F. Hagemeijer. Absorption, half-life and toxicity of oral aprindine in
    patients with acute myocardial infarction. Europ. J. Clin. Pharmacol.
    9: 21-25 (1975).
15. J.W. Ward and G.R. Kinghorn. The pharmacokinetics of disopyramide
    following myocardial infarction with special reference to oral and intra-
    venous dose regimens. J. Int. Med. Res. 4 (Suppl. 1): 49-53 (1976).
16. M. Rowland, L.Z. Benet and G.G. Graham. Clearance concepts in pharmaco-
    kinetics. J. Pharmacokin. Biopharm. 1:123-136 (1973).
17. G.R. Wilkinson. Pharmacokinetics of drug disposition: Hemodynamic con-
    siderations. Ann. Rev. Pharmacol. 15: 11-27 (1975).
18. G.R. Wilkinson and D.G. Shand. A physiological approach to hepatic drug
    clearance. Clin. Pharmacol. Therap. 18: 377-390 (1975).
19. M. Rowland. Influence of route of administration on drug availability.
    J. Pharm. Sci. 61: 70-74 (1972).
20. R.H. Cotham and D.G. Shand. Spuriously low plasma propranolol concen-
    trations resulting from blood collection methods. Clin. Pharmacol.
    Therap. 18: 535-538 (1975).
21. G.R. Wilkinson and S. Schenker. Pharmacokinetics of meperidine in man.
    Clin. Pharmacol. Therap. 19: 486-488 (1976).
22. R.A. Branch, D.G. Shand and A.S. Nies. Hemodynamic drug interactions:
    The reduction of oxyphenbutazone clearance by dl-propranolol in the dog.
    J. Pharmacol.Exptl. Therap. 187: 133-137 (1973).
23. R.W. Brauer, G.F. Leong, R.F. McElroy and R.J. Holloway. Circulatory
    pathways in the rat liver as revealed by p^{32} chromic phosphate colloid
    uptake in the isolated perfused liver preparation. Amer. J. Physiol.
    184: 593-598 (1956).

24. R.W. Brauer, R.J. Holloway and G.F. Leong. Temperature effects on radiocolloid uptake by the isolated rat liver. Amer. J. Physiol. 189: 24-30 (1957).

25. R.W. Brauer. Liver circulation and function. Physiol. Rev. 43: 115-213 (1963).

26. R.W. Brauer. Hepatic blood flow and its relation to hepatic function. Amer. J. Dig. Dis. 8: 564-576 (1963).

27. E. Engler, R.M. Nelson, H. Brown, T.W. Nielsen and S.N. Chou. Effects of changing hepatic blood flow on 17-hydroxycorticosteroid metabolism in dogs. Surgery 47: 982-986 (1960).

28. J.Y.F. Paterson and F.A. Harrison. The splanchnic hepatic uptake of cortisol in conscious and anesthetized sheep. J. Endocr. 55: 335-350 (1972).

29. T.L. Whitsett, P.G. Dayton and J.L. McNay. The effect of hepatic blood flow on the hepatic removal rate of oxyphenbutazone in the dog. J. Pharmacol. Exptl. Therap. 177: 246-255 (1971).

30. R. Nagashima and G. Levy. Effect of perfusion rate and distribution factors on drug elimination kinetics in a perfused organ system. J. Pharm. Sci. 57: 1991-1993 (1968).

31. R. Nagashima and G. Levy. Effect of flow rate on the distribution kinetics of a drug from perfusate to a perfused organ. J. Pharm. Sci. 57: 2000-2002 (1968).

32. K. Winkler, S. Keiding and N. Tygstrup. Clearance as a quantitative measure of liver function. In G. Paumgartner and R. Preisig (Eds.), The Liver: Quantitative Aspects of Structure and Function. Karger, Basel, 1973, pp 144-155.

33. R.A. Branch, A.S. Nies and D.G. Shand. The disposition of propranolol, VIII. General implications of the effects of liver blood flow on elimination from the perfused rat liver. Drug Metab. Disp. 1: 687-690 (1973).

34. D.G. Shand, D.M. Kornhauser and G.R. Wilkinson. Effects of route of administration and blood flow on hepatic drug elimination. J. Pharmacol. Exptl. Therap. 195:424-432 (1975).

35. K.S. Pang and M. Rowland. Discrimination between two models of hepatic drug clearance. In Abstracts of the Annual Meeting of the APhA Academy of Pharmaceutical Sciences, San Francisco. Vol. 5, Washington, D.C., 1975, pp 131.

36. D. Perrier and M. Gibaldi. Clearance and biologic half-life as indices of intrinsic hepatic metabolism. J. Pharmacol. Exptl. Therap. 191: 17-24 (1974).

37. L.F. Gram and J. Christiansen. First-pass metabolism of imipramine in man. Clin. Pharmacol. Therap. 17: 555-563 (1975).

38. L.F. Gram and K.F. Overo. First-pass metabolism of nortriptyline in man. Clin. Pharmacol. Therap. 18: 305-314 (1975).

39. A.C. Guyton, C.E. Jones and T.C. Coleman. Circulatory Physiology: Cardiac Output and its Regulation. Saunders, Philadelphia, Pa., 1973.

40. O.L. Wade, J.M. Bishop and K.W. Donald. Cardiac Output and Regional Blood Flow. Oxford, Blackwell, 1962.

41. P.D. Thomson, M. Rowland and K. Melmon. The influence of heart failure, liver disease and renal failure on the disposition of lidocaine in man. Amer. Heart J. 82: 417-421 (1971).

42. P.D. Thomson, K.L. Melmon, J.A. Richardson, K. Cohn, W. Steinbrunn, R. Cudihee and M. Rowland. Lidocaine pharmacokinetics in advanced heart failure, liver disease and renal failure in humans. Ann. Int. Med. 78: 499-508 (1973).

43. R.E. Stenson, R.T. Constantino and D.C. Harrison. Interrelationships of hepatic blood flow, cardiac output, and blood levels of lidocaine in man. Circulation 43: 205-211 (1971).

44. H. Halkin, P. Meffin, K. Melmon and M. Rowland. Influence of congestive heart failure on blood levels of lidocaine and its active monode-ethylated metabolite. Clin. Pharmacol. Therap. 17: 669-676 (1975).

45. C.A. Camargo., A.J. Dowdy, E.W. Hancock and J.A. Luetscher. Decreased plasma clearance and hepatic extraction of aldosterone in patients with heart failure. J. Clin. Invest. 44: 356-365 (1965).

46. N. Benowitz, R.P. Forsyth, K.L. Melmon and M. Rowland. Lidocaine disposition kinetics in monkey and man II. Effects of hemorrhage and sympathomimetic drug administration. Clin. Pharm. Therap. 16: 99-109 (1974).

47. R. Ritz, J. Cavanilles, S. Michaels, H. Shubin and M.H. Weil. Disappearance of indocyanine green during circulatory shock. Surg. Gynecol. Obstet. 136: 57-62 (1973).

48. R.A. Zito, P.R. Reid and J.A. Longstreth. Optimization of lidocaine therapy using indocyanine green clearance. Fed. Proc. 35: 222 (1976).

49. S.E. Bradley, F.J. Ingelfinger and G.P. Bradley. Hepatic circulation in cirrhosis of the liver. Circulation 5: 419-429 (1952).

50. J. Caesar, S. Shaldon, L. Chiandussi, L. Guevera and S. Sherlock. The use of indocyanine green in the measurement of hepatic blood flow and as a test of hepatic function. Clin. Sci. 21: 43-57 (1961).

51. R. Preisig, J.G. Rankin, J. Sweeting and S.E. Bradley. Hepatic hemodynamics during viral hepatitis in man. Circulation 34: 188-197 (1966).

52. P. Lundberg. Hepatic circulation during and after infectious hepatitis. Scand. J. Infect. Dis. 6: 297-304 (1974).

53. P. Lundbergh and T. Strandell. Changes in hepatic circulation at rest, during and after exercise in young males with infectious hepatitis compared with controls. Acta Med. Scand. 196: 315-325 (1974).

54. R. Groszmann, B. Kotelanski, J.N. Cohn and I.M. Khatri. Quantitation of portasystemic shunting from the splenic and mesenteric beds in alcoholic liver disease. Amer. J. Med. 53: 715-722 (1972).

55. G. Gross and C.V. Perrier. Intrahepatic portasystemic shunting in the cirrhotic patient. New Engl. J. Med. 293: 1046-1047 (1975).

56. R.A. Branch, J. James and A.E. Read. A study of the factors influencing drug disposition in chronic liver disease using the model drug (+)-propranolol. Brit. J. Clin. Pharmacol. 3: 243-249 (1976).

57. C.M. Leevy, C.L. Mendenhall, W. Leska and M.M. Howard. Estimation of hepatic blood flow with indocyanine green. J. Clin. Invest. 41: 1169-1179 (1962).

58. J.N. Cohn, I.M. Khatri, R.J. Groszmann and B. Kotelanski. Hepatic blood flow in alcoholic liver disease measured by an indicator dilution technic. Amer. J. Med. 53: 704-714 (1972).

59. R.A. Branch, J. James and A.E. Read. The clearance of antipyrine and indocyanine green in normal subjects and in patients with chronic liver disease. Clin. Pharmacol. Therap. 20: 81-89 (1976).

60. R. Gugler, P. Lain and D.L. Azarnoff. Effect of portacaval shunt on the disposition of drugs with and without first-pass effect. J. Pharmacol. Exptl. Therap. 195: 416-423 (1975).

61. D.G. Shand and R.E. Rangno. The disposition of propranolol I. Elimination during oral absorption in man. Pharmacology 7: 159-168 (1972).

62. J.W. Faigle. Blood levels of a schistosomicide in relation to liver function and side effects. Acta Pharm. Tox. 29 (Suppl 3): 233-239 (1971).

63. F.H. Messerli, J. Genest, W. Nowaczynski, O. Kuchel, M. Honda, Y. Latour and G. Dumont. Splanchnic blood flow in essential hypertension and in hypertensive patients with renal stenosis. Circulation 51: 1114-1119 (1975).

64. A.S. Nies, G.H. Evans and D.G. Shand. The hemodynamic effects of beta adrenergic blockade on the flow dependent hepatic clearance of propranolol. J. Pharmacol.Exptl. Therap. 184: 716-720 (1973).

65. A.S. Nies, G.H. Evans and D.G. Shand. Regional hemodynamic effects of beta adrenergic blockade with propranolol in the unanesthetized primate. Amer. Heart J. 85: 97-102 (1973).

66. R.A. Branch, D.G. Shand, G.R. Wilkinson and A.S. Nies. The reduction of lidocaine clearance by dl-propranolol. An example of hemodynamic drug interaction. J. Pharmacol.Exptl. Therap. 184: 515-519 (1973).

67. C.F. George, T. Fenyvesi, M.E. Conolly and C.T. Dollery. Pharmacokinetics of dextra-,laevo- and racemic propranolol in man. Europ. J. Clin. Pharmacol. 4: 74-76 (1972).

68. A.G. Bearn, B. Billing and S. Sherlock. The effect of adrenaline and noradrenaline on hepatic blood flow and splanchnic carbohydrate metabolism in man. J. Physiol. (London) 115: 430-441 (1951).

69. L.L. Cooperman. Effects of anesthetics on the splanchnic circulation. Brit. J. Anesth. 44: 967-970 (1972).

70. H.L. Price. General anesthesia and circulatory homeostasis. Physiol. Rev. 40: 187-218 (1960).

71. R.M. Epstein, S. Deutsch, L.H. Cooperman, A.J. Clement and H.L. Price. Splanchnic circulation during halothane anesthesia and hypercapnia in normal man. Anesthesiol. 27: 654-661 (1966).

72. H.L. Price, S. Deutsch, L.H. Cooperman, A.J. Clement and R.M. Epstein. Splanchnic circulation during cyclopropane anesthesia in normal man. Anesthesiol. 26: 312-319 (1965).

73. H.L. Price and A.L. Pauca. Effects of anesthesia on the peripheral circulation. Clin. Anesthesiol. 3: 73-89 (1969).

74. R.A. Branch, D.G. Shand and A.S. Nies. Increase in hepatic blood flow and d-propranolol clearance by glucagon in the monkey. J. Pharmacol. Exptl. Therap. 187: 581-587 (1973).

75. E.E. Ohnhaus. The influence of dimethylbiguanide on phenprocoumone (Marcoumar(R)) elimination. Brit. J. Clin. Pharmacol. 1: 341-342 (1974).

76. E.E. Ohnhaus, S.S. Thorgeirsson, D.S. Davies and A. Breckenridge. Changes in liver blood flow during enzyme induction. Biochem. Pharmacol. 20: 2561-2570 (1971).

77. E.E. Ohnhaus and J.T. Locher. Liver blood flow and blood volume following chronic phenobarbitone administration. Europ. J. Pharmacol. 31: 161-165 (1975).

78. R.A. Branch, D.G. Shand, G.R. Wilkinson and A.S. Nies. Increased clearance of antipyrine and d-propranolol after phenobarbital treatment in the monkey. Relative contributions of enzyme induction and increased hepatic blood flow. J. Clin. Invest. 53: 1101-1107 (1974).

79. A.S. Nies, D.G. McDevitt and G.R. Wilkinson. Effect of drug concentration and enzyme inducers on indocyanine green clearance in the rat. In Proc. 6th International Congress on Pharmacology. Helsinki, Finland, 1975, pp 384.

80. E.E. Ohnhaus and H. Siegl. Changes in renal function following chronic phenobarbitone administration. Brit. J. Pharmacol. 52: 141P (1974).

81. R.R.G. Hord, H.T. Brock, P.G. Dayton and L.I. Goldberg. Increased clearance of phenobarbital and salicylate produced by dopamine in the dog. Amer. J. Med. Sci. 258: 351-358 (1969).

82. N. Benowitz, R.F. Forsyth, K.L. Melmon and M. Rowland. Lidocaine disposition in monkey and man I. Prediction by a perfusion model. Clin. Pharmacol. Therap. 16: 87-98 (1974).

83. W.G. Crouthamel. The effect of congestive heart failure on quinidine pharmacokinetics. Amer. Heart. J. 90: 333-339 (1975).

84. B.A. Berkowitz, S.H. Ngai, J.C. Yang, J. Hempstead and S. Spector. The disposition of morphine in surgical patients. Clin. Pharmacol. Therap. 17: 629-635 (1975).

85. B. Karlen, L. Träksman and F. Sjöqvist. Decreased distribution of oxotremorine to brain after pharmacological blockade of its peripheral acetylcholine-like effects. J. Pharm. Pharmac. 23: 758-764 (1971).

32

Chapter 3

GASTROINTESTINAL ABSORPTION OF DRUGS

IN PATIENTS WITH CARDIAC FAILURE

Leslie Z. Benet, Andreas Greither and Wolfgang Meister

Most drugs taken by heart failure patients on a continuing basis are administered using the oral route. However, very few studies have been carried out to determine whether the rate and extent of absorption of these drugs is similar in heart failure patients to that noted in normal volunteers. A number of factors resulting from the disease state could cause impaired absorption of drugs in heart failure patients as listed in Table I.

Table I. Possible Factors Leading to Impaired Absorption in Heart Failure Patients

---

Pathological Changes of Intestinal Wall -

Edema of the Bowel

Decreased Splanchnic Blood Flow

Delayed Gastric Emptying

Decreased Intestinal Motility

Changes in Gastrointestinal pH

Changes in Gastrointestinal Secretions

Change in Bacterial Flora of the Gut

Drug-Drug Interactions

Firstly, pathological changes in the intestinal wall can occur in heart failure which might interfere with absorption, e.g., edema of the intestinal mucosa. This alteration has been used to explain malabsorption of fat in some patients with right-sided congestive heart failure (1,2). Berkowitz et

<u>al</u>. (1) compared the absorption of I^{131}-triolein in 25 congestive failure patients and 25 normals. Maximum blood radioactivity concentrations were significantly higher in the normal subjects than in the heart failure patients. As would be expected, a greater percentage of the total radio-active dose was found in the 48 hr fecal recovery for the heart failure patients than for normals. Figure 1 depicts the time course of radioactivity in the blood in a patient with congestive heart failure before and after treatment with diuretics. The decreased area under the curve seen before treatment with diuretics corresponds with the larger amount of radioactivity found in the 48 hr fecal samples.

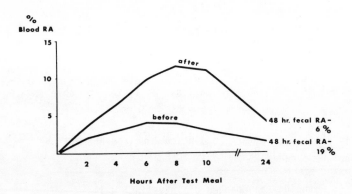

Fig. 1. Radioactive fat absorption, I^{131}-triolein, in a
congestive heart failure patient before and after
treatment with diuretics (1). (Reproduced with
permission of the publisher.)

Secondly, gastrointestinal blood flow may be the rate-limiting step in the absorption of drugs. Most drug transport has been assumed to be driven by activity gradients and to occur by passive transport mechanisms. Thus, the transfer of substances by simple diffusion across a thin membrane may be described by a useful simplification of Fick's Law as presented in Eq. 1.

$$\frac{dX_b}{dt} = P_m A_m (C_g - C_b) \qquad \text{(Eq. 1)}$$

When this equation is specifically applied to gastrointestinal absorption (3), the terms may be defined as:

X_b the amount of drug in the blood or serosal solution at any time, t

P_m the permeability coefficient for diffusion between the intestinal lumen and the blood; for a homogeneous membrane $P_m = (D_m R_{m/s})/\delta_m$

D_m the effective diffusivity of the drug in the intestinal membrane

$R_{m/s}$ the partition coefficient between membrane and solvent

δ_m the thickness of the membrane

A_m the area of membrane available for free diffusion

C_g concentration of drug in the gut or mucosal solution at any time, t

C_b concentration of drug in the blood or serosal solution at any time, t

Drugs that have crossed the intestinal epithelium are primarily removed as a function of blood flow. It can be seen in Eq. 1 that if there were no blood flow, then the concentration in the blood, C_b, would quickly approach C_g and net transfer of drug across the intestine would cease. Thus, a decreased flow may diminish the rate of removal of passively absorbed drugs (4,5). Decreased flow could possibly also interfere with active transport systems due to the reduction of the supply of oxygen to the tissues. Winne and Ochsenfahrt (5) and Winne (6) developed models and derived equations for intestinal absorption considering blood flow and counter current exchange, respectively. For the following theoretical discussion a simplified equation is presented as a modification of Eq. 1 (7):

$$\frac{dX_b}{dt} = \frac{(C_g - C_b)}{\frac{1}{P_m A_m} + \frac{1}{\alpha Q_b}} \qquad \text{(Eq. 2)}$$

where:

α fraction of blood flowing through the capillaries near the epithelium

Q_b intestinal blood flow rate

The denominator of Eq. 2 can be interpreted as the resistance of the region between the intestinal lumen and the blood pool. Winne and Remischovsky (7) have divided this resistance into two parts (first and second terms of the denominator): a.) the resistance to transport of the region between the intestinal lumen and the capillary blood (mainly the resistance of the epithelium, and b.) the resistance to drainage by blood (neglecting countercurrent exchange). Figure 2 indicates the influence of blood flow on the rate of intestinal absorption for 8 substances from the jejunum of the rat. The

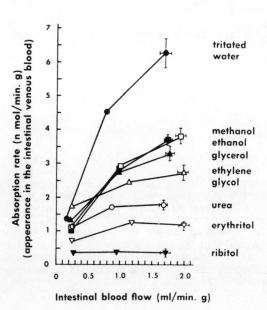

Fig. 2. Dependence of intestinal absorption on blood flow as reported by Winne and Remischovsky (7). All data corrected to a concentration of 50 n mol/ml in the solution perfusing jejunal loops of rat intestine. Bracketed points indicate 95% confidence intervals. (Reproduced with permission of the publishers.)

absorption of highly permeable materials (yielding a small term in the first part of the denominator),such as very lipid-soluble or pore diffusible substances, should be perfusion or blood flow limited. Conversely, the absorption rate of drugs characterized by low permeability of the epithelium (large first term in the denominator) may be independent of blood flow. From Fig. 2 it may be seen that the absorption of freely permeable tritiated water is very sensitive to blood flow, but that ribitol, a sugar which penetrates through epithial cells with great difficulty, is essentially unaffected by changes in intestinal blood flow in the observed range. As would be expected from Eq. 2, the absorption rate of intermediate substances such as urea appear to be flow limited at low blood flow rates but then become insensitive to blood flow at higher perfusion rates.

Winne and coworkers (4-7) have reported a blood flow dependence for a number of relatively small drug molecules. Crouthamel et al. (8) also noted a decrease in the absorption rate of sulfaethidole and haloperidol as a function of decreased mesenteric blood flow rates using an in situ canine intestinal preparation. Haass and coworkers (9) using a guinea pig model found a strong correlation between spontaneously varying portal blood flow and the amount of digitoxin and digoxin absorbed following intraduodenal infusion of the drug. As can be seen in Fig. 3, the most lipophilic of the three cardiac glycosides, i.e., digitoxin, showed the most pronounced effects as a function of blood flow. However, digoxin also showed increasing absorption rates with increasing flow. Ouabain, the most hydrophilic of the three, shows no dependence on blood flow. These results are quite consistent with the treatment of absorption rate data as predicted in Eq. 2.

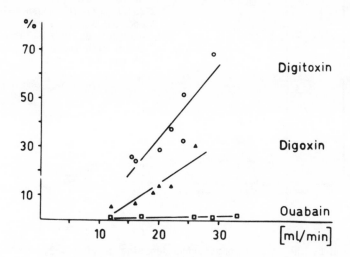

Fig. 3. Total amount of radioactivity absorbed during 1 hr, plotted versus portal blood flow (9). Ordinate: absorption as a percentage of the amount infused into the duodenum. Abscissa: mean portal blood flow in ml/min. Each point represents one guinea pig. (Reproduced with the permission of the publisher.)

Patients in heart failure would generally be expected to have a decreased output and therefore, a decreased splanchnic blood flow. This could lead to a decreased rate of absorption for compounds where blood flow rates in Eq. 2 become rate limiting. In addition, redistribution of cardiac output during cardiac failure may lead to splanchnic vasoconstriction in patients (10). This observation has recently been substantiated by experiments in the conscious dog in which an intense vasoconstriction occurred in the mesenteric beds due to acute or chronic low-output states (11). Figure 4 indicates the

37

extent to which mesenteric, renal and iliac beds respond with vasoconstriction when the low-ouput state of chronic failure was studied in conscious dogs with experimental heart failure produced by tricuspid insufficiency and pulmonary stenosis. The decreased mesenteric flow and increased resistance is of interest for this discussion.

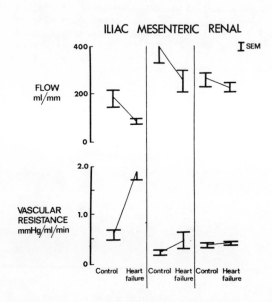

Fig. 4. Regional flows and resistances in the heart failure state compared to control values determined in the same dogs in the normal state (11). Each value indicates mean values and the standard errors in 6 conscious dogs. (Reproduced with the permission of the publisher.)

As suggested by the second term in the denominator of Eq. 2, the transport rate does not necessarily correlate directly with changes in intestinal blood flow since α, the fraction of blood flowing through the capillaries near the epithelium, may vary as a function of the pathological states causing changes in total intestinal blood flow. This is discussed in some detail by Svanvik (12) who studied the passive absorption of an easily diffusible lipid soluble substance (^{85}Kr) from the cat small intestine during various circulatory conditions. During a moderate intestinal hyperemia. induced by isoproterenol, the absorption rate of ^{85}Kr increased over that noted during the resting condition but not in direct proportion to the increase in blood flow. During a reduced perfusion pressure induced by lowering arterial inflow pressure or by raising venous outflow pressure, the absorption rate was reduced in proportion to the total intestinal blood flow. However, during the "steady state" phase of sympathetic vasoconstrictor activation, absorption rate was not reduced despite a concomitant reduction of total intestinal blood flow. In addition, Svanvik's results suggested an important function for the countercurrent diffusion exchange between ascending and descending vessels in the mucosa of the cat small intestine.

The other factors listed in Table I are not necessarily unique to changes expected for heart failure patients. The effects of delayed gastric emptying, decreased intestinal motility and changes in gastrointestinal pH have been adequately reviewed by a number of authors in terms of measurements of drug bioavailability (3,13,14). Changes in gastrointestinal secretions could lead to different degradation products and rates of degradation as well as to different volumes from which drugs may be absorbed. However, little information is available in the literature concerning affects of this nature or for the next possibility listed in Table I, changes in gut flora, which may then lead to different metabolic processes prior to absorption. The subject of drug-drug interactions has received a great deal of attention in the medical literature as reviewed recently by Koch-Weser for cardiovascular drugs (15).

Since absorption parameters must be calculated using drug levels in the plasma and urine, it is important to realize that cardiac failure may also change the drug's volume of distribution, metabolism (and thus the significance of a possible first pass effect), protein binding or renal excretion. Thereby, changes in plasma and urine levels may be produced which might not actually reflect absorption changes. As discussed in Chapter 2, a diminished volume of distribution in cardiac failure has been described for lidocaine (16), procainamide (17), and most recently quinidine (18,19).

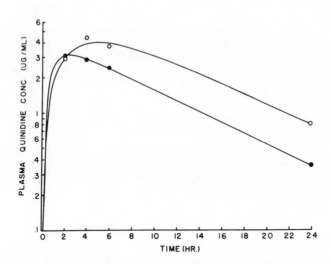

Fig. 5. Average plasma quinidine concentrations in ten normal subjects (solid circles) and ten congestive heart failure patients (unfilled circles) following oral administration of 600 mg quinidine sulfate. Data of Bellet et al. (20). Solid lines represent best computer fits of the data as reported by Crouthamel (19). (Reproduced with permission of the publisher.)

39

Figure 5 depicts average plasma quinidine concentrations in normal subjects and in congestive heart failure patients following oral administration
of 600 mg of quinidine sulfate. The smooth lines drawn through the points
were based on calculations performed by Crouthamel (18,19) for data previously published by Bellet et al. (20). Crouthamel suggests that congestive
heart failure reduces the rate and amount of quinidine absorption following
oral dosing as well as reducing the volume of distribution. However, no
changes in the elimination rate were noted when congestive heart failure
patients were compared to normals. Analysis of this data requires that the
investigator be aware of changes in disposition parameters for quinidine when
attempting to evaluate the absorption characteristic. Even though the data
points plotted in Fig. 5 are the average values for ten subjects and measurements are only available at four time points, two conclusions seem justified:
a.) the time for peak following oral dosing in congestive heart failure
patients is to the right of that seen in normals, and b.) blood levels in the
heart failure patients are greater than those seen for normals at the 4, 6
and 24 hr time points. It is important to realize that the time to peak
would shift to the right as a result of either a decreased elimination rate
for the drug or a decreased absorption rate. In the published analysis of
the data (19) Crouthamel reports elimination half-lives of 6.5 and 6.7 hrs
in the normal and heart failure patients respectively. Thus, the change in
peak time can logically be attributed to a decreased rate of absorption in
the heart failure patients. (Our analysis of the data indicates an average
half life of 8.0 hrs in the heart failure patients, but we would also calculate a decreased rate of absorption in the patients.) The hypothesized
change in the extent of absorption (18,19) is questionable since this analysis was made by comparing the amount of unchanged quinidine appearing in the
urine. Although congestive heart failure patients excreted amounts of unchanged drug which were less than half that seen in normals (see Table II),
creatinine clearances in congestive heart failure patients were also less
than half the value found in normals. For a drug which is both metabolized
and excreted unmetabolized in the urine, changes in the percent of drug excreted unmetabolized may be expected to reflect changes in creatinine clearance without implying any change in the extent of absorption.

Table II. Oral Quinidine (600 mg) in Normals And
Congestive Heart Failure Patients[a]

Subjects	Amount Excreted Unchanged in 24 Hrs	Creatinine Clearance
Normal	129.3 mg	109 ml/min
Heart Failure	56.6 mg	51 ml/min

[a]After Bellet et al. (20).

Thus, in the data discussed above, it is probable that the extent of availability is the same or less for congestive heart failure patients as compared to normals. Therefore, the suggested decrease in the volume of distribution for quinidine in heart failure patients is probably correct, even though intravenous studies have not been carried out to substantiate this. This hypothesized decreased volume of distribution in heart failure patients is consistent with the results previously reported for lidocaine and procainamide (16,17).

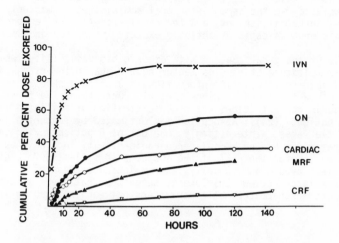

Fig. 6. Cumulative excretion of metolazone and metabolites in urine after intravenous or oral dose of 2.5 mg ^{14}C-metolazone. IVN, intravenous administration to normal subjects; ON, oral administration to normal subjects; CARDIAC, oral administration to patients with cardiac insufficiency; MRF, oral administration to patients with mild renal failure; CRF, oral administration to patients with chronic renal failure (21). (Reproduced with the permission of the publisher.)

A limited amount of data has appeared in the literature indicating that the extent of absorption of drugs may be reduced in congestive heart failure patients. Figure 6 depicts the cumulative excretion of metolazone, a recently introduced substituted quinazoline sulfonamide with diuretic activity, after doses of the radio-labelled drug to normal subjects by the intravenous route and to normal subjects, patients with cardiac insufficiency, patients with mild renal failure and patients with chronic renal failure by the oral route (21). A decreased total extent absorbed in cardiac patients may be implied from the figure. Koch-Weser (17,22) has indicated that procainamide absorption may be decreased in patients with cardiac problems. In fasting normal subjects, procainamide is rapidly absorbed from the GI tract, peak serum concentrations are achieved within one hour and absorption under such conditions is reasonably complete. However, in patients with acute myocardial infarction intestinal absorption is generally markedly delayed. No detectable amount of procainamide may appear in the serum for two hours after ingestion and peak concentration may not be reached until the fifth hour. Occasionally, patients absorb less than 50% of the oral dose and reach therapeutic plasma concentrations only when the oral dose is greatly increased or when the drug is administered parenterally. In 1961, Anderson and coworkers (23) studied the absorption of hydrochlorothiazide in three subjects with congestive heart failure. In these patients the maximum concentration of hydrochlorothiazide in the serum after oral administration was only one half that obtained in normal persons, and the renal excretion of radioactivity was lower for this drug which is essentially excreted unchanged in humans.

In spite of the great concern with digoxin bioavailability, which has resulted in a multitude of studies measuring the absorption of the drug from commercial dosage forms, little information is available about absorption in patients with heart failure. Doherty et al. contributed the first measurements of digoxin concentrations after administration of tritiated digoxin in solution to patients (24). Absorption was estimated by measuring the radioactivity in the feces. Interestingly, one out of 5 patients with cardiac failure excreted 45% of the administered radioactivity in 5 days as opposed to an averaged 15% for the rest of the subjects (4 patients, 2 "controls"). The same patient needed an unusually large maintenance dose of 1.0 mg digoxin per day. In a later review (25) Doherty suggested that there were no apparent differences in pharmacokinetic parameters between individuals in conges-

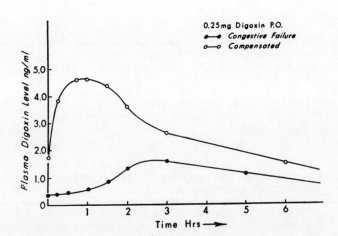

Fig. 7. Serum digoxin levels achieved during and after clearing of congestive failure in an 85 pound female patient as reported by Oliver et al. (27). (Reproduced with the permission of the publisher.)

42

tive heart failure compared with those who were not. The cardiology textbook by Hurst and Logue (26) makes the following statement:

> When digoxin is given orally, the desired clinical effect may not be achieved in some patients unless large amounts are administered. The majority of such patients will respond, when average doses of the drug are given in the muscle or vein rather than orally. This suggests that in some patients with heart failure the absorption of digoxin may be greatly decreased.

Oliver et al. (27) compared postabsorptive digoxin levels in three patients while in congestive failure and later after congestive failure had disappeared. Figure 7 depicts the results obtained in one of the subjects. While in congestive heart failure, there is a very slow increase in serum digoxin levels until a peak value is reached at three hours. However, in the same patient given an identical dose of digoxin after congestive heart failure had cleared, there is a prompt, marked increase in digoxin levels to significantly higher concentrations. In a second patient differences in levels are significantly different during the first two hours following dosing. However, serum levels are then approximately similar for the next ten hours, indicating that the effective levels of the drug in the postabsorptive phase were not markedly influenced by congestive heart failure. In a third patient experiencing only mild congestive failure very little difference is observed at any time.

Recently Ohnhaus et al. (28) investigated digoxin absorption in 7 patients with severe right-sided heart failure. Tritiated solution and one commercial tablet were given before and after successful treatment. Blood and urine digoxin concentrations were estimated by liquid scintillation counting and radioimmunoassay. Pharmacokinetic analysis, based upon computation of parameters using plasma-level time concentrations and cumulative urinary excretion, revealed no differences between noncompensated and compensated states. Since the study involved only oral doses, no estimates of volume of distribution, total body clearance and absolute bioavailability could be made. Comparing the cumulative excretion of tritiated digoxin in 120 hrs, average values of 50.2 and 47.7% of dose were found in noncompensated and compensated patients respectively. Assuming that the fraction of the dose excreted unmetabolized remained constant and that the percentage of excreted labelled metabolites is negligible, this result does suggest that absorption of digoxin solution was not influenced by the degree of cardiac failure. The results for the commercial tablet assayed using radioimmunoassay techniques are consistent with the solution results but appear questionable. Ohnhaus et al. (28) found that 24.6 and 30.9% of the tablet were excreted in 24 hrs for the noncompensated and compensated states respectively. Since the patients were on maintenance therapy, one would expect the 24 hr excretion of unchanged drug to be approximately 1.6 to 2 times that observed by the investigators assuming the preparation studied had the average bioavailability of 65% and the fraction to be excreted unmetabolized was 80% (25).

Although there is evidence of impaired absorption for most drugs studied, we feel that the studies discussed above are inconclusive, because they do not fulfill one or more of the following criteria, which we believe necessary for adequate studies on drug absorption in cardiac failure:

a.) Cardiac failure may not only affect gastrointestinal absorption, but may also lead to changes in distribution, metabolism and excretion of drugs (as discussed in Chapter 2). Therefore, disposition characteristics have to be investigated in order to define input characteristics without ambiguity.
b.) The patient group has to be clinically described and should include a reasonable number of subjects.
c.) In making comparisons properly matched control groups have to be selected. Neglecting age, for example, may preclude meaningful interpretations because this variable may considerably affect pharmacokinetics, as recently reviewed by Triggs and Nation (29).

We have recently studied the pharmacokinetics and diuretic effect of furosemide in congestive heart failure patients (30). Furosemide is one of the more potent diuretics available and one of those most frequently used in treating congestive heart failure and other forms of fluid retention. Most clinicians, however, have experienced the unpredictability of its diuretic activity; some patients responding promptly and vigorously to small oral doses, others requiring rather massive intravenous amounts of drug in order to achieve a diuresis. Six males and one female patient between 45 and 75 years of age and weighing from 62-93 kg were studied. The patients experienced moderate to severe congestive heart failure related to cardiomyopathy or coronary disease and all but one were in a compensated status without apparent edema. The renal function and plasma electrolyte values were ostensibly normal in each case and all the patients had previously been on furosemide for at least four weeks so that the dose expected to provoke an appropriate diuretic response was known. Each patient received randomly intravenous or oral furosemide on alternate days in doses of 40, 80 or 120 mg (according to the patient's previous treatment). Blood samples were collected at frequent intervals for 8 hrs and urine samples were collected at time of voiding up to 24 hrs. The plasma drug assay was performed using a spectroflurometric method, sensitive to variations of 0.1 mcg/ml in the range of 0.5 - 5 mcg/ml. Although the fluorometric method is not entirely specific, recent work has shown that the principle metabolite detected by this method is found in the urine rather than the plasma.

Figure 8 depicts the plasma concentration-time curve following oral and intravenous administration of 120 mg of furosemide in a patient, S.S., with severe congestive heart failure and moderate edema. The curves are representative of those seen for each of the patients; the intravenous route of administration yields initially higher levels of the drug, but in the slow disposition phase (beta phase), the disappearance half-life is essentially the same for the oral and intravenous routes of administration. The following pharmacokinetic parameters (mean ± SD) were determined for the seven patients: $\alpha = 0.093 \pm 0.053$ min^{-1}; $\beta = 0.016 \pm 0.005$ min^{-1}; $t_{\frac{1}{2}\beta} = 76.7 \pm 30.6$ min; volume of the central compartment as a percent of body weight = $7.10 \pm 1.38\%$; volume of distribution at steady state as a percent of total body weight = $11.4 \pm 1.6\%$; total body clearance as a fraction of body weight = 1.48 ± 0.35 ml/min/kg. The small volume of distribution found in these subjects is consistent with a highly protein bound drug which is ionized at plasma pH. The volume of distribution at steady state as a fraction of total body weight is almost identical to previously reported volumes in normal subjects (31) and to volumes calculated from the data in normals by Rupp and

44

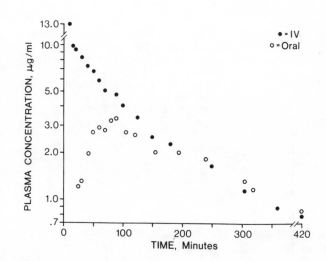

Fig. 8. Plasma concentration-time curves following oral (open circles) and intravenous (solid circles) administration of 120 mg furosemide to patient S.S. (30).

Hajdu (32). There is apparently no significant decrease in the volume of distribution due to congestive heart failure. No change would be expected for a drug which remains essentially in the central comparment. For drugs such as lidocaine, the volume of distribution decreases when cardiac output decreases (Chapter 2). However, for furosemide where little peripheral distribution is seen, decreased cardiac output apparently has no effect on the volume of distribution. The total body clearance and rate constants for elimination found in this study were significantly lower than those reported in normals by Cutler et al. (31) and Kelly et al. (33). However, the half life for elimination reported here is similar to more recent values reported by Beermann and coworkers in normal subjects (34) and the average clearance reported here is almost identical to that calculated from the values in normals reported by Rupp and Hajdu (32).

Figure 9 compares the range and average extent of availability found in our study (30) with data reported in normals by Kelly et al. (33). In our study availability measurements ranged from 0.34 to 0.80 with an average of 0.61 ± 0.16. This average is almost identical to the 0.65 ± 0.25 value reported by Kelly et al. (33), the 0.65 value reported by Beermann and co-workers (34), and the 0.58 value of Rupp and Hajdu (32). It is of interest to note that the patient with severe congestive heart failure and moderate edema, whose plasma level values are depicted in Fig. 8, had an availability of 0.60. Although the total amount of urine eliminated in a 24 hr period following oral and intravenous dosing did not correlate with differences in availability, an apparent relation was found with the ratio of urine flow rates, oral to intravenous, when cumulative flows are calculated at corresponding times 3-4 hrs postdosing, i.e., during the time interval where significant blood levels may be measured. This is consistent with the results of Rupp and Hajdu (32) who demonstrated a good correlation between furosemide

45

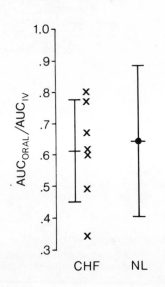

FUROSEMIDE AVAILABILITY

Fig. 9. Comparison of the mean
and range for the extent of
oral availability found by
Greither et al. (30) in 7
congestive heart failure
patients (CHF) and by Kelly
et al. (33) in 4 normals
(NL).

serum concentrations and urine flow rates for both oral and intravenous
doses. The ratio of urine flow rates oral to intravenous ranged from 0.55 to
0.79 with an average of 0.67 ± 0.09.

Lag times before measureable drug was absorbed as well as absorption
rates varied markedly from subject to subject and did not correlate with the
extent of oral availability. Figure 10 depicts a graph of the percent of
drug remaining to be absorbed as a function of time, calculated by the method
of Loo and Riegelman (35), for the subject showing the lowest extent of oral
availability. No absorption of the drug takes place for a 40 min period;
thereafter, the drug is absorbed quite rapidly by an apparent first order
process with a half life of 13 min. In contrast, another subject whose absorption profile is depicted in Fig. 11 had a 12 min lag time and then begins to
absorb drug at a first order rate with a half life of about 29 min. However,
at a point where approximately 35% of the drug remains to be absorbed, the
first order absorption process is interrupted and from then on there is dis-
continuity in absorption with an obvious slowing of the absorption rate.
Lag times average 28 ± 15 min and varied from 10-47 min in these fasted
subjects. Time to peak ranged from 50-150 min with a mean of 86 min.

The following conclusions can be made concerning the pharmacokinetics of
absorption and elimination of furosemide in patients with congestive heart
failure (30): a.) The absorption may be delayed with a lag time before

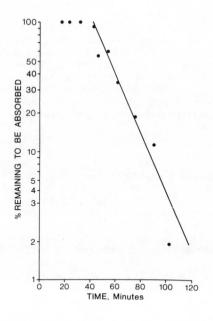

Fig. 10. Semilogarithmic plot
of percent drug remaining to
be absorbed versus time for
subject J.C. following a 40 mg
oral dose of furosemide. A
40 min lag time is observed
before absorption begins.
However, the drug is then
absorbed quite rapidly by an
apparent first order process
with a half-life of 13 min.

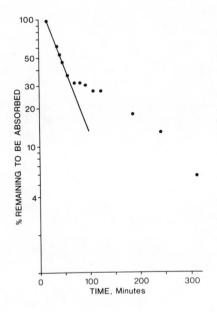

Fig. 11. Semilogarithmic plot
of percent of drug remaining
to be absorbed versus time for
subject F.H. following an
80 mg oral dose of furosemide.
See text for further explanation.

47

appearance in the plasma; this most likely being due to variable rates of gastric emptying. Absorption then proceeds at different rates in different individuals; the amount of drug orally absorbed is incomplete and the absorption process is often erratic. However, the variation in the extent of absorption noted in these seven congestive heart failure patients are similar to values reported in normals. b.) The volume of distribution for furosemide, in contrast to certain other pharmacologic agents, is not diminished in congestive heart failure. c.) There is an apparent relation between the ratio of areas under the curve oral to intravenous and the ratio of diuretic response during the time interval where measureable plasma concentrations are observed.

Summary

A number of pathophysiological factors may cause impaired drug absorption in cardiac failure. Two of them, gastrointestinal edema and especially decreased mesenteric blood flow, are discussed in some detail. Studies of absorption with quinidine, procainamide, hydrochlorothiazide, metolazone and digoxin are evaluated. They suggest impaired absorption of quinidine, procainamide, hydrochlorothiazide and metolazone, but studies with digoxin are contradictory. As cardiac failure may also lead to changes in distribution, metabolism and excretion of drugs, and as these factors have not been adequately investigated in these studies, the interpretations remain inconclusive. The pharmacokinetics of furosemide appear to be unchanged in cardiac failure.

Acknowledgments

Studies in the authors' laboratories were supported in part by National Institutes of Health Grant No. GM-16496. During the course of this work Dr. Meister was supported as a Fellow of the Paul Martini-Stiftung. The authors express their appreciation to Drs. Keith Cohn, Steven Goldman and John S. Edelen, our collaborators in the furosemide studies discussed here, for allowing us to abstract portions of that work. Finally, the authors wish to thank Ms. Linda Kiefer for her invaluable help in preparing the manuscript and figures and for serving as the medium of contact between Europe and San Francisco.

References

1. D. Berkowitz, M. N. Croll and W. Likoff. Malabsorption as a complication of congestive heart failure. Am. J. Cardiol. 11: 43-47 (1963).
2. J. Hakkila, T. E. Mäkelä and P. I. Halonen. Absorption of I^{131} triolein in congestive heart failure. Am. J. Cardiol. 5: 295-299 (1960).
3. L. Z. Benet. Biopharmaceutics as a basis for the design of drug products. In E. J. Ariëns (ed.), Drug Design, Volume IV, Academic Press, New York, 1973, pp. 1-35.
4. L. Ther and D. Winne. Drug absorption. Ann. Rev. Pharmacol. 11: 57-70 (1971).
5. D. Winne and H. Ochsenfahrt. Die formale Kinetik der Resorption unter Berücksichtigung der Darmdurchblutung. J. Theoret. Biol. 14: 293-315 (1967).
6. D. Winne. The influence of villous counter current exchange on intestinal absorption. J. Theor. Biol. 53: 145-176 (1975).
7. D. Winne and J. Remischovsky. Intestinal blood flow and absorption of non-dissociable substances. J. Pharm. Pharmac. 22: 640-641 (1970).
8. W. G. Crouthamel, L. Diamond, L. W. Dittert and J. T. Doluisio. Drug absorption VII: Influence of mesenteric blood flow on intestinal drug absorption in dogs. J. Pharm. Sci. 64: 661-671 (1975).
9. A. Haass, H. Lüllmann and T. Peters. Absorption rates of some cardiac glycosides and portal blood flow. Europ. J. Pharmacol. 19: 366-370 (1972).
10. J. Ferrer, S. E. Bradley, H. O. Wheeler, Y. Enson, R. Preisig and R. M. Harvey. The effect of digoxin in the splanchnic circulation in ventricular failure. Circulation 32: 524-537 (1965).
11. C. B. Higgins, S. F. Vatner, D. Franklin and E. Braunwald. Pattern of differential vasoconstriction in response to acute and chronic low-output states in the conscious dog. Cardiovasc. Res. 8: 92-98 (1974).
12. J. Svanvik. Mucosal blood circulation and its influence on passive absorption in the small intestine: An experimental study in the cat. Acta Physiol. Scand., Suppl.385: 1-44 (1973).
13. G. Levy. Biopharmaceutical considerations in dosage form design and evaluation. In J. B. Sprowls, Jr. (ed.), Prescription Pharmacy, 2nd Edition, Lippincott, Philadelphia, 1970, pp. 36-102.
14. M. Gibaldi. Introduction to Biopharmaceutics. Lea and Febiger, Philadelphia, 1970.
15. J. Koch-Weser. Drug interactions in cardiovascular therapy. Am. Heart J. 90: 93-116 (1975).
16. P. D. Thomson, K. L. Melmon, J. A. Richardson, K. Cohn, W. Teinbrunn, R. Cudihee and M. Rowland. Lidocaine pharmacokinetics in advanced heart failure, liver disease and renal failure in humans. Ann. Intern. Med. 78: 499-508 (1973).
17. J. Koch-Weser and J. W. Klein. Procainamide dosage schedules, plasma concentrations, and clinical effects. JAMA 215: 1454-1460 (1971).
18. W. G. Crouthamel. Elimination of quinidine in congestive heart failure. NEJM 290: 1379-1380 (1974).
19. W. G. Crouthamel. The effect of congestive heart failure on quinidine pharmacokinetics. Am. Heart J. 90: 335-339 (1975).
20. S. Bellet, L. R. Roman and A. Boza. Relation between serum quinidine levels and renal function. Am. J. Cardiol. 27: 368-371 (1971).

21. W. J. Tilstone, H. Dargie, E. N. Dargie, H. G. Morgan and A. C. Kennedy. Pharmacokinetics of metolazone in normal subjects and in patients with cardiac or renal failure. Clin. Pharmacol. Ther. 16: 322-329 (1974).

22. J. Koch-Weser. Pharmacokinetics of procainamide in man. Ann. N.Y. Acad. Sci. 179: 370-382 (1971).

23. K. V. Anderson, H. R. Brettell and J. K. Aikawa. C^{14}-labelled hydrochlorothiazide in human beings. Arch. Intern. Med. 107: 168-174 (1961).

24. J. E. Doherty, W. H. Perkins and G. K. Mitchell. Tritiated digoxin. Studies in human subjects. Arch. Intern. Med. 108: 531-539 (1961).

25. J. E. Doherty. The clinical pharmacology of digitalis glycosides: A review. Am. J. Med. Sci. 255: 382-414 (1968).

26. J. W. Hurst and R. B. Logue. Treatment of heart failure. In J. W. Hurst and R. B. Logue (eds.), The Heart, Arteries and Veins, 2nd Edition, McGraw Hill, New York, 1970, p. 462.

27. G. C. Oliver, R. Tazman and R. Frederickson. Influence of congestive heart failure on digoxin level. In O. Storstein (ed.), Symposium on Digitalis, Gyldenal Norsk Forlag, Oslo, Norway, 1973, pp. 336-347.

28. E. E. Ohnhaus, S. Vozeh and E. Nüesch. Untersuchungen zur Resorption von Digoxin bei Patienten mit dekompensierter Rechtsherzinsuffizienz. Schweiz. med. Wschr. 105: 1782-1783 (1975).

29. E. J. Triggs and R. L. Nation. Pharmacokinetics in the aged: A review. J. Pharmacokin. Biopharm. 3: 387-418 (1975).

30. A. Greither, S. Goldman, J. S. Edelen, K. Cohn and L. Z. Benet. Erratic and incomplete absorption of furosemide in congestive heart failure. Am. J. Cardiol. 37: 139 (1976).

31. R. E. Cutler, A. W. Forrey, T. G. Christopher and B. M. Kimpel. Pharmacokinetics of furosemide in normal subjects and functionally anephric patients. Clin. Pharmacol. Ther. 15: 588-596 (1974).

32. W. Rupp and P. Hajdu. Pharmacokinetics and pharmacodynamics of a diuretic agent. In H. J. Dengler (ed.), Symposium on Pharmacological and Clinical Significance of Pharmacokinetics, F. K. Schattauer Verlag, Stuttgart, 1970, pp. 105-111.

33. M. R. Kelly, R. E. Cutler, A. W. Forrey and B. M. Kimpel. Pharmacokinetics of orally administered furosemide. Clin. Pharmacol. Ther. 15: 178-186 (1974).

34. B. Beermann, E. Dahlen, B. Lindstrom and A. Rosen. On the fate of furosemide in man. Europ. J. Clin. Pharmacol. 9: 57-61 (1975).

35. J. C. K. Loo and S. Riegelman. New method for calculating the intrinsic absorption rate of drugs. J. Pharm. Sci. 57: 918-928 (1968).

II. HEPATIC AND
METABOLIC FUNCTION

Chapter 4

PHARMACOKINETICS IN DISEASE STATES

MODIFYING HEPATIC AND METABOLIC FUNCTION

Malcolm Rowland, Terrence F. Blaschke, Peter J. Meffin

and Roger L. Williams.

As the liver is the major site for drug metabolism, an impression
evails that special care should be taken in administering drugs to
tients with disease states modifying hepatic and metabolic function.
jective data, mostly obtained in patients with hepatic disorders, while
nerally supporting this impression, are limited and appear in conflict.
is conflict was evident in some of the earlier studies; the elimination
lf-lives ($t_{\frac{1}{2}}$) for aminopyrine, antipyrine, dicoumarol, salicylic acid (1),
lbutamide (2) and phenylbutazone (3), were found to lie within the range
und in healthy subjects, while those for chloramphenicol (4) and isoniazid
) were prolonged.   In many of these earlier studies the analytical
ecificity is questionable.   But this inconsistency in the changes of the
armacokinetics of a drug in patients with liver disorders still persists in
e more recent studies, (Table I), that use specific assays.   The apparent
nflict arises from an attempt to make simple generalisations about an
tremely complex situation.   The liver performs a multiplicity of functions,
cluding the elimination of drugs by metabolism and biliary excretion.
tabolic pathways, each with a different set of co-factor requirements, are
merous and the contribution of any pathway to total elimination varies with
e drug.   Disorders of the liver, local or diffuse, are caused by many
seases; each disease affects the various levels of hepatic organisation to
different extent.   Genetics, other drugs and the duration of disease
rther complicate the situation.   In this review, an attempt is made to
itically examine the influence of altered hepatic and metabolic function on
e pharmacokinetic parameters of various drugs; no attempt has been made to
mprehensively survey the literature.   The implications of alterations in
e pharmacokinetic parameters in drug therapy are explored.

TABLE I.	CHANGES IN TOTAL PLASMA CLEARANCE AND	
DISEASE	DECREASED CLEARANCE INCREASED HALF-LIFE	
Cirrhosis	Ampicillin - Lewis and Jusko, 1975 (6) Amobarbital - Mawer, et al, 1972 (7) Antipyrine - Branch, et al, 1973 (8) Chloramphenicol - Kunin, et al, 1959 (4)[a] Diazepam - Klotz, et al, 1975 (9) Isoniazid - Levi, et al, 1968 (5)[a] Lidocaine - Thomson, et al, 1973 (10) Meperidine - Klotz, et al, 1974 (11) Phenobarbital - Alvin, et al, 1975 (12)[a] Phenylbutazone - Levi, et al, 1968 (5)[a]	
Acute Viral Hepatitis	Antipyrine - Branch, et al, 1973 (8) Diazepam - Klotz, et al, 1973 (9) Hexobarbital - Breimer, et al, 1975 (13)[c] Meperidine - McHorse, et al, 1975 (14)	
Chronic Active Hepatitis	Antipyrine - Branch, et al, 1973 (8) Diazepam - Klotz, et al, 1975 (9)	
Obstructive Jaundice	Antipyrine - Branch, et al, 1973 (8)	

[a] Half-life only measured
[b] Total blood clearance
[c] Horizontal study

Unravelling The Facts

Classification of the Disease

Table I lists the change in the half-life, and where measured, total (plasma)clearance of a number of drugs in patients with liver disease. Grouped together there appears to be no consistent relationship between disease and drug handling with almost as many drugs showing no change as those showing a decrease; only with tolbutamide does total clearance increase.

ELIMINATION HALF-LIFE OF SOME DRUGS IN LIVER DISEASE

UNCHANGED	INCREASED CLEARANCE DECREASED HALF-LIFE
Tolbutamide - Nelson, 1964 (2)[a]	
Lidocaine - Williams,et al,1976 (15)[b,c] Phenobarbital - Alvin,et al,1975 (12)[a] Phenylbutazone - Levi,et al,1968 (5)[a] Phenytoin - Blaschke, et al, 1975 (16)[c] Warfarin - Williams, et al, 1976 (17)[c]	Tolbutamide - Held,et al,1976 (18)[a] Tolbutamide - Williams,et al,1976 (19)[c]

When, however, liver disease is divided into chronic (especially cirrhosis) and acute and reversible situations, for example, acute viral hepatitis, a clearer picture emerges. With the exception of tolbutamide, there is a decreased total clearance of all drugs measured in cirrhosis; no increased total clearance of a drug has been reported in cirrhotic patients. In contrast, in acute viral hepatitis, there appears to be a fairly even division between those drugs in which a decreased total clearance, or an increased half-life, has been reported and those where no change could be detected. With one drug, tolbutamide, an increased total clearance was noted. What little data exists, appears to suggest that drug elimination may be diminished in chronic active hepatitis and obstructive jaundice.

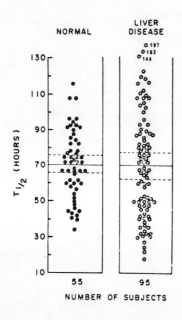

Fig. 1. Phenylbutazone half-lives in
normal subjects and in patients with liver disease (5).
(Reproduced with permission
of the publisher).

The failure of some earlier workers to demonstrate an effect of liver disease on drug metabolism may be due to the co-administration of other drugs. For example, a comparison study by Levi, et al, (5), of phenylbutazone half-lives in normal subjects and patients with liver disease, revealed no differences between the two groups, except for a greater variability in the half-life amongst the patients in the liver disease group (Figure 1). When, however, both groups of patients were further sub-divided on the basis of whether they received other drugs, a much clearer picture emerged (Figure 2). In subjects not receiving other drugs, phenylbutazone was handled more slowly in patients with liver disease than in normal subjects. Evidently some of the drugs received induce the enzymes responsible for phenylbutazone elimination. Certainly, phenobarbital and prednisone, both enzyme-inducing agents, diminished the antipyrine half-life in patients with chronic active hepatitis (8). Drugs, then, can obscure the influence of hepatic dysfunction on pharmacokinetics. So too can genetic factors.

Many metabolic pathways are under genetic control and when metabolism is a major route of elimination, inter-subject variability in the pharmacokinetics of a drug in the normal population may be wide. Levi, for example, found over a two-fold variation in the half-life of phenylbutazone in normal individuals without drugs (Figure 2) and an even wider variation in the half-life of other drugs in healthy individuals has been reported (20). Such wide inter-subject variability makes changes in the pharmacokinetics of a drug difficult to detect. This is particularly so when studying the effect of

56

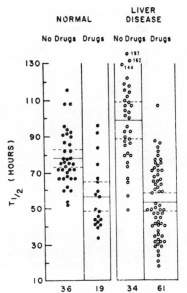

Fig. 2. Influence of drug treatment on phenylbutazone half-lives in normal subjects and in patients with liver diseases (5). (Reproduced with permission of the publisher).

chronic disease on pharmacokinetics; assessment is usually made by comparing drug handling in the patient population with its handling in an otherwise comparable population without the disease. Then, unless the sample size is large (to permit a reasonable estimate of the population mean) and the influence of the disease on drug handling consistent, a difference between the two populations may fail to be detected when one exists. Conversely, a difference in drug kinetics between a small group of patients and controls, might suggest an influence of disease when none exists.

In reversible hepatic diseases, such as acute viral hepatitis, genetic and environmental factors may be eliminated with a longitudinal study in which the kinetics of a drug are studied in the individual, during, and after, recovery from the disease; each person acts as his own control. This longitudinal design enables the influence of the disease on pharmacokinetics to be assessed using only a small sample size. Williams, et al, (19), for example, showed in a relatively small population that, although the tolbutamide half-life differed between subjects, there was consistent decrease in the elimination half-life of this drug during acute viral hepatitis (Figure 3).

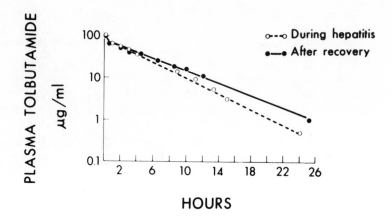

Fig. 3.   Accelerated elimination of tolbutamide in a patient
during the acute phase of viral hepatitis (19).

Pharmacokinetic Parameters

The blood or plasma half-life of a drug has been the parameter most
frequently used to compare its handling in hepatic disease.   The half-life,
however, is controlled by two potentially independent parameters; the volume
of distribution (V) and the total clearance (CL_T) of the drug

$$t_{\frac{1}{2}} = \frac{0 \cdot 693 V}{CL_T} \qquad \text{(Eq. 1)}$$

An alteration in distribution may partially or totally explain a change in
half-life.   Clearance is therefore the preferred index for measuring the
efficiency with which the elimination organs remove a drug (21, 22).

To ascertain the volume of distribution and the clearance, a drug should
be given either intravenously or parenterally to ensure full availability
into the systemic circulation.   Unfortunately, in most studies, the drug was
given orally, thereby complicating the interpretation.   In some of the few
studies where drug was given parenterally, the volume of distribution remained
unaltered in liver disease (Table II), and any change in half-life can be
ascribed to a change in total clearance.   Nonetheless, the potential for
misinterpreting the mechanism for a change in half-life does exist.   Indeed,
part of the prolongation in the half-life of ampicillin, diazepam and lidocaine in cirrhosis is caused by an increased volume of distribution.

TABLE II.   CHANGES IN THE VOLUME OF DISTRIBUTION OF SOME DRUGS IN LIVER DISEASE

Drug	Disease	Volume of Distribution[a] (L/Kg)		Comment[c]	Reference
		In Health	In Liver Disease		
Ampicillin	Cirrhosis	0.28(0.07)[d]	0.84(0.61)	Increased	Lewis and Jusko, 1975 (6)
Amobarbital	Cirrhosis	0.97(0.29)	1.46(0.30)	Increased	Mawer, et al, 1972 (7)
Diazepam	Cirrhosis	1.13(0.28)	1.74(0.21)	Increased	Klotz, et al, 1975 (9)
Hexobarbital	Acute Viral Hepatitis	1.10(0.12)	1.10(0.40)	Unchanged	Briemer, et al, 1975 (13)
Lidocaine	Cirrhosis	1.3 (0.35)	2.3 (0.96)	Increased	Thomson, et al, 1974 (10)
Lidocaine	Acute Viral Hepatitis[b]	2.0 (0.5)	3.1 (1.8)	Unchanged	Williams, et al, 1976 (15)
Meperidine	Cirrhosis	4.17(1.33)	5.76(2.55)	Unchanged	Klotz, et al, 1975 (11)
Meperidine	Acute Viral Hepatitis	5.56(1.80)	5.94(2.65)	Unchanged	McHorse, et al, 1975 (14)
Phenytoin	Acute Viral Hepatitis[b]	0.64(0.06)	0.68(0.04)	Unchanged	Blaschke, et al, 1975 (16)
Tolbutamide	Acute Viral Hepatitis[b]	0.15(0.03)	0.15(0.03)	Unchanged	Williams, et al, 1976 (19)
Warfarin	Acute Viral Hepatitis[b]	0.21(0.02)	0.19(0.04)	Unchanged	Williams, et al, 1976 (17)

a.   Volume of distribution at steady state (Vd_{SS}).

b.   Horizontal study: In health refers to patients in recovery phase of study.

c.   The volume of distribution is considered unchanged if in the t-test p>0.05.

d.   Standard deviation in parenthesis.

Distribution can also change with age.   Essentially all the increase in the
half-life of diazepam with age (20-80 yr) in healthy volunteers is associated
with an increased volume of distribution (9).   And, since patients with
chronic liver disorders are often middle-aged, the control subjects must be
age matched.

Clearance: Total clearance (usually assessed by dividing an intravenous
bolus dose by the total area under the blood or plasma concentration time
curve (21)) is an average value and it is the sum of the clearance by each
elimination organ, usually the liver and the kidney.   Total clearance must
be divided into its component parts before any assessment of the influence
of hepatic and renal dysfunction can be fully ascertained.   This point was
admirably illustrated by Lewis and Jusko (6).   They showed that the absence
of a change in the total plasma clearance of ampicillin in cirrhosis arose
because a decrease in the renal clearance was compensated for by an increase
in the hepatic clearance of this antibiotic (Figure 4).   They adequately
accounted for the lower renal clearance of ampicillin in the cirrhotic subjects; these subjects were older than the normal volunteers used as the
control and renal function is known to diminish with age (23).   They failed,
however, to explain the much higher hepatic clearance of ampicillin in the
cirrhotic patients.

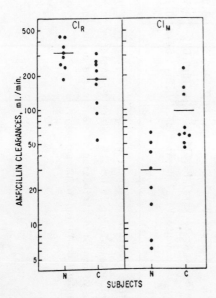

Fig. 4.   Comparison of the renal clearance and non-renal (hepatic)
clearance of ampicillin between
normal (N) and cirrhotic (C)
subjects.   The horizontal line
represents the average values
(6).   (Reproduced with permission of the publisher).

1 some instances it may even be necessary to sub-divide the hepatic clear-
nce into biliary clearance and the clearance associated with each metabolic
athway of the drug.   This would arise when there is a selective effect on a
articular metabolic process which may not (if it is   minor) be detected by
easuring changes in total clearance.   To define the clearance associated
ith a particular metabolic pathway, the formation of the metabolite must be
easured and this would be warranted when the metabolite contributes signifi-
antly to the pharmacologic effect, or is toxic.

The cause for a change in hepatic clearance (CL_H) may be several fold.
easured directly across the liver, hepatic clearance is the product of
epatic blood flow (Q) and the extraction ratio (E) of the compound by the
iver

$$CL_H = Q.E. \qquad \text{(Eq. 2)}$$

lood flow and extraction ratio appear to be independent parameters control-
ing clearance.   But much experimental evidence suggests otherwise; the
xtraction ratio decreases with increasing blood flow.   While our under-
tanding of the factors affecting hepatic clearance is incomplete, the
esults of one model (22), for which there is some supportive evidence (24,
5), indicate that (26)

$$CL_H = Q \left[\frac{f\ CL_{int}}{Q + f\ CL_{int}} \right] \qquad \text{(Eq. 3)}$$

hus, not only is the extraction ratio dependent upon blood flow (Q) but it
s also dependent upon the fraction of drug in blood unbound (f) and the
ntrinsic metabolic clearance of this drug (CL_{int}).   The intrinsic clearance
ay be regarded as the clearance of a drug when there are no flow limitations.
t is a measure of the hepatocellular metabolic activity and it is related to
he maximum velocity (Vm) and the Michealis-Menten constant (Km) of each
nzyme system associated with hepatic removal by

$$CL_{int} = \sum_{i=1}^{n} \frac{Vm_i}{Km_i + C_{u,L}} \qquad \text{(Eq. 4)}$$

$_{u,L}$ being the concentration of unbound drug surrounding the hepatic enzymes.
his model of hepatic clearance assumes that the unbound drug in blood leaving
he liver equals $C_{u,L}$.

. Clearance and Flow: According to this model and other models (27) of
epatic clearance, for drugs with an extraction ratio approaching unity
$CL_{int} \gg Q$), organ clearance ($CL \approx Q$) is very sensitive to changes in liver
lood flow, essentially independent of blood binding and only marginally
ensitive to changes in hepatic drug metabolising activity.

Table III lists examples of compounds highly cleared by the liver. Besides the direct effect on the clearance of these well extracted drugs, a disturbed hepatic perfusion (often seen in cirrhosis) could also diminish the elimination of those drugs whose metabolism is rate limited by oxygen; included might be drugs undergoing microsomal oxidation. In acute viral hepatitis, liver blood flow may be increased (28) and so might therefore the clearance of well extracted drugs. The failure to find such a change with lidocaine (a well extracted drug) would then imply that its hepatic extraction ratio and hence intrinsic metabolic clearance is reduced in this disease (15).

TABLE III.   SOME COMPOUNDS KNOWN TO BE, OR SUSPECTED OF BEING, HIGHLY EXTRACTED BY THE LIVER IN MAN.

Acetylsalicylic Acid	Lidocaine
Aldosterone	Meperidine
Alprenolol	Morphine
Desmethylimipramine	Nortriptyline
Isoproterenol	Organic Nitrates
	Pentazocine

---

b. Clearance and Binding: Most drugs are predominantly metabolised but poorly extracted by the liver (E<0.2).   An examination of Equation 3 shows that for poorly extracted drugs ($Q>CL_{int}$), blood clearance ($CL=f\ CL_{int}$) and plasma clearance ($CL=f_p CL_{int}$; where f_p is the fraction of drug in plasma unbound) are not limited by perfusion but are limited by the hepatic enzymatic activity and the binding of drug in blood (and plasma).

Drug binding is sometimes altered in liver disease and a failure to appreciate the role of binding on the clearance of a poorly extracted drug can lead to incorrect conclusions.   Williams, et al, (19), for example, noted a consistent shortening of the half-life of tolbutamide during acute viral hepatitis (Figure 3).   As the volume of distribution remained unchanged (Table II), an elevated total (predominantly hepatic) plasma clearance of this poorly extracted drug during the acute phase of the disease is inferred.   But, contrary to initial appearances, hepatocellular enzyme activity is unchanged.   It happens that the plasma binding of tolbutamide is also decreased and when corrections were made for these differences in binding the clearance based on unbound drug remained unchanged in all subjects during, and after recovery from,the disease (Table IV).   The same events are seen with phenytoin but to a lesser extent.   What causes the decreased binding of these drugs is uncertain.   (The reader may also wish to refer to Chapter 9, where changes in binding for phenytoin in hypoalbuminemic subjects are likewise shown to not cause changes of intrinsic clearance).   Phenytoin and tolbutamide are acidic drugs and are primarily bound to albumin in plasma; but in acute viral hepatitis, plasma albumin levels are unchanged.   An elevated bilirubin, associated with this disease, is a partial explanation;

bilirubin added to recovery phase plasma, at the same concentration found in patients during the acute phase, decreased the plasma binding of tolbutamide but not to the same extent as seen in vivo. (Further discussion of binding in hyperbilirubinemia may be found in Chapter 9). Perhaps other displacing agents are present in plasma, or the affinity between drug and albumin decreases during acute hepatitis.

Altered plasma binding can also mask the effects of chronic liver disease on drug metabolism. Thus, although the total (primarily hepatic) plasma clearance of amobarbital, a poorly extracted drug, is essentially unaltered, its intrinsic clearance, reflecting hepatic drug metabolising activity, is significantly depressed in patients with chronic liver disease and hypoalbuminaemia (Table IV). Here, a low serum albumin, reflecting a

TABLE IV.	CHANGES IN PLASMA CLEARANCE, PLASMA BINDING AND INTRINSIC CLEARANCE OF SOME POORLY EXTRACTED DRUGS DURING LIVER DISEASE				
Drug	Condition	Plasma Clearance (mls/hr/Kg)	Fraction Drug in Plasma Unbound	Intrinsic Clearance (mls/hr/Kg)	Reference
Amobarbital	Healthy	34	0.39	88	Mawer, et al, 1972 (7)
	Chronic Liver Disease Group I. (>3G% albumin)	42	0.40	104	
	Group II. (<3G% albumin)	28	0.69	38	
Tolbutamide	Control Phase	18	0.060	300	Williams,et al 1976 (17)
	Acute Viral Hepatitis	26	0.10	260	
Phenytoin	Control Phase	1.9	0.097	19	Blaschke,et al 1975 (16)
	Acute Viral Hepatitis	2.2	0.130	17	

sustained depression of protein synthesis, produces a predictable fall in the binding of this drug (and others bound to albumin) which in turn tends to offset the depressed metabolic activity. Interestingly, in cases of mild liver disease, where serum albumin is normal, both plasma binding and intrinsic clearance of amobarbital are within the normal range (Group I, Table IV). (A lower plasma binding could also explain the elevated metabolic plasma clearance of ampicillin in cirrhosis; the intrinsic metabolic clearance may be unchanged).

Distribution: As total plasma (or blood) clearance can mask an effect on the drug metabolising activity (CL_{int}), so the volume of distribution (based on plasma or blood) can mask changes in drug distribution.   For example, no change was found in the volume of distribution (based on plasma) of phenytoin and tolbutamide in acute viral hepatitis (Table II) and yet there were accompanying decreases in the plasma binding of both drugs (16, 19).   A diminished plasma binding is normally associated with an increased volume of distribution and a failure to note such a change automatically implies that drug tissue binding must also have diminished.   Perhaps bilirubin, which is partially responsible for the diminished binding in plasma, also causes part, if not all, of the diminished tissue binding of these drugs.   The result of reduced plasma and tissue binding is an increase in the unbound concentration for a given amount of drug in the body.   For phenytoin and tolbutamide calculations, assuming that the unbound drug distributes evenly throughout total body water spaces, indicate that the percent unbound drug in the body will increase by approximately 10 percent.   This increase is inconsequential in drug therapy but it may be greater for other drugs and should always be considered.

Amobarbital and ampicillin are acids and both bind to albumin.   The volume of distribution, based on plasma and blood, is also increased in severe chronic liver disease (Table IV).   With amobarbital, the increase is entirely explained by a low serum albumin; the volume of distribution based on unbound drug in healthy volunteers and those with severe liver disease are similar (7).   This may also be so for ampicillin and perhaps all other drugs bound to albumin.   A depressed albumin may not lead to corresponding increases in the volume of distribution of amines; many of these are substantially bound to plasma constituents other than albumin (29).

Absorption: Studies of the influence of altered hepatic and metabolic function on oral drug absorption are few and complicated by the need to ascertain the clearance of the drug at the time of measurement.   Preferably, the comparison should be made between the extent of absorption, or absolute availability (F), in the same individual in health and disease.   With reversible   liver disease this may be possible; with chronic disease, comparison is made between a population of healthy subjects and patients. Absolute availability is usually measured by comparing the total area under the plasma (blood) concentration time curve $[\int_0^\infty Cdt]$, or the cumulative amount of drug excreted unchanged $[Ae_\infty]$ following oral and intravenous administration of the drug

$$F_{oral} \quad = \quad CL_T \cdot \frac{\left[\int_0^\infty Cdt\right]_{oral}}{Dose_{oral}} \qquad (Eq. 4)$$

$$CL_T \quad = \quad \frac{Dose_{iv}}{\left[\int_0^\infty Cdt\right]_{iv}} \qquad (Eq. 5)$$

64

$$F_{oral} = \frac{[Ae_{\infty}]_{oral}}{f_e Dose_{oral}} \qquad (Eq.\ 6)$$

$$f_e = \frac{[Ae_{\infty}]_{iv}}{Dose_{iv}} \qquad (Eq.\ 7)$$

where f_e is the ratio of renal to total clearance. In the calculations of F, it is assumed that clearance and f_e, determined intravenously, are the same as when the drug is given orally. In a healthy subject, this assumption is reasonable. It may be invalid in the sick; the disease state changes with time and even giving the oral and intravenous dose at different times of the same day may not suffice. If a change in the elimination half-life was noted between the two treatments, then attempting to correct the area for this change in the elimination rate constant (30) may still be invalid if part of the change was caused by altered drug distribution. A possible solution might be to simultaneously give a heavy labelled isotope of a drug intravenously and the drug orally and so, by using mass-spectrographic techniques, resolve the situation. This stable isotope technique is being increasingly employed in pharmacokinetics.

When the drug can only be given orally, there is no unambiguous method for assessing a change in absorption in disease. A difference in area between healthy and sick subjects could be due to either a change in absorption, clearance, or both. The situation cannot be resolved further.

All material absorbed from the gastrointestinal tract passes through the liver before entering the general circulation. Any drug, therefore, that is highly extracted by the liver has a low oral availability; the phenomenon is commonly known as "the first-pass effect". Examples are propranolol, lidocaine, nortriptyline. How well the drug traverses the liver is primarily a function of the hepatocellular activity. When this activity is depressed, the availability of these highly cleared compounds should be increased. Portal bypass, which can occur in cirrhosis, should also result in an enhanced availability of highly cleared compounds; this has been demonstrated experimentally (31) and no doubt occurs clinically. (See Chapter 2 for discussion of flow changes on the extent of availability and Chapter 5 for further treatment of portal bypass).

Correlation with Liver Function Tests: Attempts to correlate changes in the pharmacokinetics (especially hepatic clearance) of drugs with various liver function tests have been generally unsuccessful. Liver function tests include serum total bilirubin, albumin, glutamic oxalacetic transaminase(SGOT), glutamic pyruvate transaminase (SGPT), lactic dehydrogenase (LDH) and alkaline phosphatase. This failure to find a correlate contrasts with the successful use of creatinine clearance to reflect the renal clearance of drugs in patients with impaired renal function. (See Chapter 10. A discussion of the influence of kidney disease on drug metabolism is also included in Chapter 10).

In chronic liver disease, serum albumin might serve as a crude index of hepatic drug metabolising activity. Patients with a depressed serum albumin (<3gm %) show a prolonged half-life of antipyrine, a drug essentially unbound and predominantly cleared by the liver (8), a depressed intrinsic clearance of amobarbital (7) and a diminished N-demethylation of aminopyrine (32). It has been suggested that a low albumin reflects a depressed synthesis of hepatic proteins including those involved with drug metabolism. The shortening of the antipyrine half-life in patients when given phenobarbital, an agent known to increase the amount of microsomal enzymes (33), favours this hypothesis. So does the correlation of a depressed clearance of both antipyrine (a lowly cleared drug) and indocyanine green (a highly cleared drug) with a decreased serum albumin and prolongation in the prothrombin index (34). (See Chapter 5 for further discussion).

In acute viral hepatitis, the situation is less clearly defined. A diminished clearance of indocyanine green, which consistently occurred, is not always parallelled by a decrease in antipyrine clearance (Williams, personal communication), nor is the diminished indocyanine green clearance always matched by a parallel decrease in the clearance of lidocaine, another highly cleared and presumably flow dependent drug (15). Moreover, while the clearances of indocyanine green, antipyrine, diazepam and hexobarbital are depressed, the intrinsic clearances of tolbutamide, phenytoin and warfarin remained unchanged (Table V). With the exception of indocyanine green, which is excreted unchanged into the bile, all these compounds are eliminated primarily by oxidation. These data suggest that the sensitivity of the various oxidative pathways to acute hepatic insult differ. They also suggest that changes in the clearance of antipyrine, which has been considered as a model drug to reflect abnormalities in microsomal drug metabolism, may prove of limited or no value for predicting changes in clearance of other drugs. Indeed, it is difficult to envisage that any single compound could be used to reflect the complex changes that occur in altered hepatic function.

Therapeutic Consequences - A Working Hypothesis

Whether an alteration in the pharmacokinetics of a drug has any therapeutic consequence depends on several factors. One is the change in the unbound, and presumably pharmacologically active, drug concentration; another is the response to a given unbound drug concentration. It is well to remember the latter. For example, changes in the clotting system and not in its pharmacokinetics explains the increased prothrombin time to a dose of warfarin during the acute phase of viral hepatitis (Figure 5). In the subsequent analysis, however, it is assumed that the responsiveness to a given unbound drug concentration is unaffected by disease and that any metabolite is inactive and non-toxic.

66

TABLE V. CHANGES IN THE INTRINSIC METABOLIC CLEARANCE OF SEVERAL DRUGS, PRIMARILY OXIDISED, IN ACUTE VIRAL HEPATITIS

DRUG	STRUCTURE	MAJOR PRIMARY OXIDATION PRODUCT	INTRINSIC METABOLIC CLEARANCE	REFERENCE
TOLBUTAMIDE			UNCHANGED	Williams, et al, 1976 (19)
PHENYTOIN			UNCHANGED	Blaschke, et al, 1975 (16)
WARFARIN			UNCHANGED	Williams, et al, 1976 (17)
ANTIPYRINE			DECREASED	Branch, et al 1973 (8)
DIAZEPAM			DECREASED	Klotz, et al, 1975 (9)
HEXOBARBITAL			DECREASED	Breimer, et al, 1975 (13)

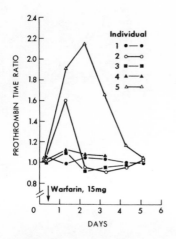

Fig. 5. Changes in the prothrombin time ratio following the administration of a small oral dose (15 mg) of racemic warfarin to patients during the acute phase of viral hepatitis (17). (Reproduced with permission of the publisher).

In therapeutics, four general situations can be envisaged; the drug is given as a single intravenous (or parenteral) dose; the drug is given as a single oral dose; the drug is given as a constant intravenous (or parenteral) infusion, or an oral dose is given chronically. To consider the likely outcome to a change in a pharmacokinetic parameter in each of these four situations, a relationship must be established between clearance, organ blood flow, binding of drug in plasma (and blood) and drug metabolising activity. For this purpose, it is assumed that the relationship between these variables is adequately expressed by Equation 3. To the extent that the model of hepatic clearance, upon which Equation 3 is based, is not fully proven, the conclusion drawn below are to be considered as guidelines rather than definitive statements.

Intravenous Bolus Dose: The maximum intensity of pharmacologic effect following a given dose of drug is unlikely to change significantly. Thus, although the volume of distribution (based on plasma or blood) may substantially increase in hepatic dysfunction (Table II), the volume of distribution based on unbound drug only changes minimally. The duration of effect will therefore only increase with an increase in the area under the unbound drug concentration time curve ($Area_{unbound}$). Following an intravenous bolus dose, the total area under the blood level time curve is given by

$$Area_{blood} = \frac{Dose}{CL_T} \qquad\qquad (Eq.\ 8)$$

When all the drug is cleared by the liver, then, by appropriate substitution for total clearance from Equation 3 into Equation 8, one obtains

$$\text{Area}_{\text{unbound}} = \frac{f \cdot \text{Dose}}{Q\left[\dfrac{f\ \text{CL}_{\text{int}}}{Q + f\ \text{CL}_{\text{int}}}\right]} \qquad\text{(Eq. 9)}$$

For a highly cleared drug ($Q < \text{CL}_{\text{int}}$), the above equation reduces to

$$\text{Area}_{\text{unbound}} = f\ \frac{\text{Dose}}{Q} \qquad\text{(Eq. 10)}$$

whereas for poorly cleared compounds ($Q > \text{CL}_{\text{int}}$) the resulting equation is

$$\text{Area}_{\text{unbound}} = \frac{\text{Dose}}{\text{CL}_{\text{int}}} \qquad\text{(Eq. 11)}$$

Several conclusions emerge from the relationships above. For a highly cleared drug, the duration of effect should be sensitive to changes in hepatic blood flow and binding of drug to components in blood but only marginally sensitive to changes in hepatocellular enzymatic activity. For a lowly cleared drug, the duration of effect should only be sensitive to changes in the intrinsic metabolic clearance of the drug; a diminished binding alone may increase the volume of distribution but, because clearance is also increased, the half-life of drug (bound and unbound) remains essentially unchanged.

Single Oral Dose: The general equation relating drug availability (F) to the area under the blood level time curve following a single oral dose is

$$\text{F Dose} = \text{CL}_T \text{Area}_{\text{blood}} \qquad\text{(Eq. 12)}$$

For drugs exclusively eliminated by the liver and in which the sole cause for a low oral availability is the first-pass effect ($F = 1-E$), then substitution for F and clearance from Equation 3 into Equation 12 gives (22, 35)

$$\text{Area} = \frac{\text{Dose}}{f\ \text{CL}_{\text{int}}} \qquad\text{(Eq. 13)}$$

and the area under the unbound plasma concentration ($\text{Area}_{\text{unbound}}$) is given by (26)

$$\text{Area}_\text{unbound} = \frac{\text{Dose}}{CL_\text{int}} \qquad \text{(Eq. 14)}$$

Thus, while changes in hepatic blood flow can influence the clearance and the availability of a highly extracted compound, irrespective of how well it is cleared, the area under the blood level time curve following oral drug administration is independent of hepatic blood flow. And the area under the unbound level time curve is independent of either hepatic blood flow or binding changes. For all drugs, only changes in the drug metabolising activity (CL_int) will produce (proportional) changes in the unbound plasma concentration time curve. Viewed differently, if one can exclude the possibility of loss due to either formulation effects, instability in the luminal content, or gut wall metabolism, then a change in the area under the unbound curve following oral drug administration is an accurate reflection of a change in the drug metabolising system.

Although the relationship between area under the unbound concentration curve and the various pharmacokinetic parameters following oral drug administration is relatively simple, the relationship between these variables and the intensity and the duration of pharmacologic effect is complex. Generally, a diminished intrinsic clearance will result in some increase in the intensity and a more prolonged response, but it would be relatively uncommon for these changes in response to be sufficiently great to warrant a reduced single oral dose.

Constant Intravenous Infusion

The relationship between the steady state blood level (C_{ss}), steady state concentration of the unbound drug ($C_{u,ss}$) and the constant rate of infusion (R^O) is defined by

$$C_{ss} = \frac{R^O}{CL_T} = \frac{R^O}{Q\left[\dfrac{f\ CL_\text{int}}{Q + f\ CL_\text{int}}\right]} \qquad \text{(Eq. 15)}$$

$$C_{u,ss} = f\ C_{ss} = \frac{f\ R^O}{Q\left[\dfrac{f\ CL_\text{int}}{Q + f\ CL_\text{int}}\right]} \qquad \text{(Eq. 16)}$$

The similarity between the above equations and those for the area under the curve following an i.v. bolus dose is apparent and the conclusions are the same. For highly cleared compounds, the unbound concentration will be elevated when either hepatic blood flow is depressed or binding is diminished. For lowly cleared drugs, the unbound steady state concentration is only sensitive to changes in the drug metabolising activity and although altered binding will alter the blood concentration, the unbound steady state drug concentration should remain the same. Whether the half-life, and hence the time to reach the plateau (36), changes, depend upon the relative changes in the total clearance and the volume of distribution of the drug.

Chronic Oral Dosing

This is the most prevalent situation in therapeutics; the aims are usually to maintain a constant concentration of unbound drug for the period of treatment. In this situation, a dose is given at intervals of time τ, and the average blood concentration at the plateau ($\overline{C}_{ss}$) is defined by (37)

$$\overline{C}_{ss} = \frac{F \cdot Dose}{CL_T \cdot \tau} \qquad \text{(Eq. 17)}$$

If all the drug administered reaches the liver, and the liver is the sole eliminating organ, then substitution from Equation 3 for $F(= 1-E)$ and CL_T into the above equation leads to the following

$$\overline{C}_{ss} = \frac{Dose}{f \ CL_{int}\tau} \qquad \text{(Eq. 18)}$$

$$\overline{C}_{u,ss} = \frac{Dose}{CL_{int} \cdot \tau} \qquad \text{(Eq. 19)}$$

The similarity of the steady state equations following multiple oral dose therapy to the area under the curve following single dose therapy is immediately apparent and the conclusions are the same. For all drugs, whether highly or poorly cleared, the steady state blood concentration depends on binding and intrinsic clearance; it should be independent of blood flow. And, more importantly, for all drugs, the unbound concentration at steady state should depend solely on the drug metabolism activity of the liver; it should be independent of hepatic blood flow and binding. Thus, a diminished intrinsic clearance of a drug may require a reduction in its dosage regimen; a diminished blood flow or binding should not. Stated differently, in practice, all changes in the pharmacokinetics of a drug are secondary to changes in its intrinsic clearance. (Levy, in Chapter 9, comments on the variability in peak and valley free concentration values where binding changes but average blood concentrations of free drug remain constant).

71

Capacity Limited Elimination

Changes in the intrinsic clearance can result from either a change in V_m or K_m of the enzyme system(s). If the hypothesis, that in liver disease the diminished activity is due to a depressed protein synthesis (8), then V_m and not K_m will be diminished. For many drugs, in the therapeutic plasma concentration range, the kinetics are independent of concentration ($C < K_m$), and under these conditions, changes in V_m will produce proportional changes in CL_{int} and hence in the steady state unbound drug concentration following chronic oral therapy. The change in the steady state unbound concentration with changes in V_m will be much more dramatic, however, if elimination in the therapeutic concentration range is characterised by Michealis-Menten kinetics (for example, phenytoin (38)). Under these circumstances, the intrinsic clearance is given by

$$CL_{int} = \frac{V_m}{K_m + \bar{C}_{u,ss}} \qquad (Eq.\ 20)$$

which, when substituted into Equation 19 and appropriately rearranged, reduces to

$$\bar{C}_{u,ss} = \frac{K_m\ R^o}{V_m - R^o} \qquad (Eq.\ 21)$$

Here, we see that if the rate of administration, R^o (Dose/τ) approaches V_m, then even if V_m changes only 10 percent, for example, dramatic increases in the unbound concentration of the drug at steady state will result. This capacity limited elimination may explain the extremely high steady state plasma concentration of phenytoin in a patient with hepatic disease receiving normal doses of this drug (39).

Concluding Remarks

The pharmacokinetics of many drugs are altered in diseases involving modified hepatic and metabolic function, but only when the intrinsic metabolic clearance is reduced would a modification in chronic oral dosage regimens seem warranted. Even then, adjustments in dosage would only seem reasonable when the usual regimen results in the unbound drug concentration at the plateau approaching or exceeding the upper limit of the therapeutic range. Hence primarily concern for adjustment is with drugs having a narrow therapeutic index. These drugs are also ones where drug level monitoring is appropriate.

The conclusions made regarding the influence of changes in blood flow, binding and hepatocellular activity were based on a model of hepatic clearance which needs further evaluation and on the assumption that the liver was the sole clearing organ. In situations where renal function plays a more predominant role, the change in liver function will have less effect on the plasma concentration time profiles.   In patients with portal-systemic shunts, drugs highly extracted by the liver are more available and dosage of such drugs in these patients may need to be reduced.

At this (data gathering) stage, it is difficult to discern any clear methods for predicting the dose requirements for a patient with a given degree of a specific liver disease.   More fundamental knowledge is required of the pathways of drug metabolism, the co-factor requirements and the relationship of these to hepatic dysfunction.   The pharmacokinetic models will need to be continually refined and evaluated in the pathological states before they will become of any predictive value.

The absence of a change in the pharmacokinetic parameters of a drug with altered hepatic function does not exclude the need to modify its regimen. Patients, for example, in acute viral hepatitis, respond excessively to the standard doses of warfarin, despite no significant change in its pharmacokinetics.   Such an observation stresses the need to place pharmacokinetic data into a broader therapeutic framework.

Acknowledgments

The work reported by the authors which eminated from their activities was supported in part by National Institute of Health, Grants GM.16496, GM.01791 and GM.00001, and N.I.H. Training Grant, GM.00725-13.

References

1.   B.B. Brodie, J.J. Burns and M. Weiner. Metabolism of drugs in subjects with Laennec's cirrhosis. Med. Exp. (Basel), 1: 290-292 (1959).

2.   E. Nelson.   Rate of metabolism of tolbutamide in test subjects with liver disease or with impaired renal function. Amer.J. Med. Sci. 248: 657-659 (1964).

3.   M. Weiner, T. Chenkin and J.J. Burns.   Observations on the metabolic transformation and effects of phenylbutazone in subjects with hepatic disease. Amer.J. Med. Sci. 228: 36-39 (1954).

4.   C.M. Kunin, A.J. Glazko and M. Finland. Persistence of antibiotics in blood of patients with acute renal failure. II. Chloramphenicol and its metabolic products in the blood of patients with severe renal disease or hepatic cirrhosis. J. Clin. Invest. 38: 1498-1508 (1959).

5.   A.J. Levi, S. Sherlock and D. Walker. Phenylbutazone and isoniazid metabolism in patients with liver disease in relation to previous drug therapy. Lancet. 1: 1275-1279 (1968).

6. G.P. Lewis and W.J. Jusko. Pharmacokinetics of ampicillin in cirrhosis. Clin. Pharmacol. Therap. 18: 475-484 (1975).
7. G.E. Mawer, N.E. Miller and L.A. Turnberg. Metabolism of amylobarbitone in patients with chronic liver disease. Br.J. Pharmacol. 44:549-560(1972)
8. R.A. Branch, C.M. Herbert and A.E. Read. Determinants of serum antipyrine half-lives in patients with liver disease. Gut. 14: 569-573 (1973).
9. U. Klotz, G.R. Avant, A. Hoyumpa, S. Schenker and G.R. Wilkinson. The effects of age and liver disease on the disposition and elimination of diazepam in adult man. J. Clin. Invest. 55: 347-359 (1975).
10. P.D. Thomson, K.L. Melmon, J.A. Richardson, K. Cohn, W. Steinbrunn, R. Cudihee and M. Rowland. Lidocaine pharmacokinetics in advanced heart failure, liver disease, and renal failure in humans. Ann. Intern. Med. 78: 499-508 (1973).
11. U. Klotz, T.S. McHorse, G.R. Wilkinson and S. Schenker. The effect of cirrhosis on the disposition and elimination of meperidine (pethidine) in man. Clin. Pharmacol. Ther. 16: 667-675 (1974).
12. J. Alvin, T.S. McHorse, A. Hoyumpa, M.T. Bush and S. Schenker. The effect of liver disease in man on the disposition of phenobarbital. J. Pharm. Exp. Therap. 192: 224-235 (1975).
13. D.D. Breimer, W. Zilly and E. Richter. Pharmacokinetics of hexobarbital in acute hepatitis and after apparent recovery. Clin. Pharmacol. Therap. 18: 433-440 (1975).
14. T.S. McHorse, G.R. Wilkinson, R.F. Johnson and S. Schenker. Effect of acute viral hepatitis in man on the disposition and elimination of meperidine. Gastroenterology. 68: 775-780 (1975).
15. R.L. Williams, T.F. Blaschke, P.J. Meffin, K.L. Melmon and M. Rowland. Influence of viral hepatitis on the disposition of two compounds with high hepatic clearance: lidocaine and indocyanine green. Clin. Pharmacol. Therap. In press.
16. T.F. Blaschke, P.J. Meffin, K.L. Melmon and M. Rowland. Influence of acute viral hepatitis on phenytoin kinetics and protein binding. Clin. Pharmacol. Therap. 17: 685-691 (1975).
17. R.L. Williams, W.L. Schary, T.F. Blaschke, P.J. Meffin, K.L. Melmon and M. Rowland. The influence of acute viral hepatitis on the disposition and pharmacologic effect of warfarin. Clin. Pharmacol. Therap. In press.
18. V.H. Held, R. Elsert and H.F.V. Oldershausen. Pharmacokinetics of glymidine (glycodiazine) and tolbutamide in acute and chronic liver disease. Arzneim. Forsch. 23: 1801-1807 (1973).
19. R.L. Williams, T.F. Blaschke, P.J. Meffin, K.L. Melmon and M. Rowland. The influence of acute viral hepatitis on the disposition and plasma binding of tolbutamide. In press.
20. A.H. Conney, B. Craver, R. Kuntzman and E.J. Pantuck. Drug metabolism in normal and disease states. In T. Teorell, R.L. Dedrick and P.G. Condliffe (eds), Pharmacology and Pharmacokinetics, Plenum Press, New York, 1973, pp. 147-162.
21. M. Rowland. Influence of route of administration on availability. J. Pharm. Sci. 61: 70-74 (1972).
22. M. Rowland, L.Z. Benet and G.G. Graham. Clearance concepts in pharmacokinetics. J. Pharmacokin. Biopharm. 1: 123-136 (1973).
23. K. Siersbaek-Nielsen, J.M. Hansen, J. Kampmann and M. Kristensen. Rapid evaluation of creatinine clearance. Lancet. 1: 1133-1134 (1971).
24. K.S. Pang and M. Rowland. Hepatic clearance of drugs: Discrimination between two models. In Abstracts of the 16th National Meeting of the APhA Academy of Pharmaceutical Sciences, San Francisco, Vol.2, Washington

D.C. 1975.
25. D.G. Shand, D.M. Kornhauser and G.R. Wilkinson. Effects of route of administration and blood flow on hepatic drug elimination. J. Pharmacol. Exp. Therap. 195: 424-432 (1975).
26. G.R. Wilkinson and D.G. Shand. A physiological approach to hepatic drug clearance. Clin. Pharmacol. Therap. 18: 377-390 (1975).
27. K. Winkler, S. Keiding and N. Tygstrup. Clearance as a quantitative measure of liver function. In The Liver: Quantitative aspect of structure and function, Karger-Basel, 1973, pp. 144-155.
28. P. Lundberg. Hepatic circulation in hepatitis. Acta Med. Scand. (Suppl), 563: 7-56 (1974).
29. G.J. Tucker, R.N. Boyes, P.O. Bridenbaugh and D.C. Moore. Binding of anilide-type local anesthetics in human plasma. I. Relationships between binding, physicochemical properties and anesthetic activity. Anesthesiology, 33: 287-303 (1970).
30. J.G. Wagner. Biopharmaceutics and relevant pharmacokinetics. Drug Intelligence Publications, Hamilton, Illinois, 1971, pp.182-183.
31. R. Gugler, P. Lain and D.L. Azarnoff. Effect of portacaval shunt on the disposition of drugs with and without first-pass effect. J. Pharmacol. Exp. Therap. 195: 416-423 (1975).
32. G.W. Hepner and E.S. Vessel. Quantitative assessment of hepatic function by breath analysis after oral administration of ^{14}C aminopyrine. Ann. Int. Med. 83: 632-638 (1975).
33. A.H. Conney, C. Davison, R. Gastel and J.J. Burns. Adaptive increases in drug-metabolising enzymes induced by phenobarbital and other drugs. J. Pharmacol. Exp. Ther. 130: 1-8 (1960).
34. R.A. Branch, J.A. James and A.E. Read. Major determinants of drug disposition in chronic liver disease: A study with indocyanine green and antipyrine. Br.J. Clin. Pharmacol. 2: 370P-371P (1975).
35. D. Perrier and M. Gibaldi. Clearance and biological half-life as indices of intrinsic hepatic metabolism. J. Pharmacol. Exp. Ther. 191: 17-24 (1974)
36. M. Rowland. Drug administration and regimens. In, K.L. Melmon and H.F. Morrelli (eds), Clinical Pharmacology and Therapeutics. Macmillan, New York, 1971, pp.21-60.
37. J.G. Wagner, J.I. Northam, C.D. Alway and O.S. Carpenter. Blood levels of drug at the equilibrium state after multiple dosing. Nature (Lond.) 207: 1301-1302 (1965).
38. N. Gerber and J.G. Wagner. Explanation of dose-dependent decline of diphenylhydantoin plasma levels by fitting to the integrated form of the Michaelis-Menten equation. Res.Comm.Chem.Path.Pharma. 3: 455-466 (1972).
39. H. Kutt, W. Winters, R. Scherman and R. McDowell. Diphenyl-hydantoin and phenobarbital toxicity. The role of liver disease. Arch. Neurol. 11: 649-656 (1964).

Chapter 5

HEPATIC DRUG CLEARANCE IN CHRONIC LIVER DISEASE

Robert A. Branch and David G. Shand

Introduction

The pharmacokinetics of drugs that are eliminated by the liver can be quantitatively explained on a physiological basis from a knowledge of the effects of four biological determinants a) the activity of the drug metabolizing enzymes or intrinsic hepatic clearance for free drug (CL_{int} as defined in Chapter 4), b) hepatic blood flow, c) drug binding and d) the anatomical arrangement of the hepatic circulation (1,2 and Chapters 2 and 4 of this book). In discussing the effects of hepatic blood flow on drug clearance, the action of the enzymes must be expressed in terms of total drug in blood. In this chapter we have therefore used the term intrinsic clearance with reference to total drug, that is the clearance of drug from liver water multiplied by the free fraction of drug in blood (CL_{int} f according to Chapter 4). Disturbances of all the determinants of hepatic elimination can occur in chronic liver disease and result in predictable changes in drug disposition.

The liver has a limited repertoire of responses to pathological insults, with the result that chronic liver disease tends to present a similar pathophysiological and clinical picture irrespective of etiology. Although the etiological agent will determine the rate of progression of the disease process, the natural history of chronic liver disease is a tendency to progression, with the life expectancy of patients being considerably reduced. A combination of cell injury followed by fibrosis and hepatocyte regeneration results in a marked derangement of the normal hepatic architecture. The cells that are not involved in disease processes appear to be morphologically normal, and normal concentrations of the mixed function oxidase enzymes responsible for the metabolism of many drugs have been found in the early stages of the development of cirrhosis (3,4). The finely balanced blood supply from the splanchnic capillary bed via the portal vein and from the hepatic artery to the portal area is disturbed, as is the passage of blood from the center of the hepatic acinus through the sinusoids between parenchyma cells to the hepatic vein. As the disease progresses there is gross distortion with loss of the tributaries of the portal vein and viable hepatocytes regenerate to form islands of hepatic parenchyma which are thought to be only perfused by hepatic artery. At the same time, direct portal tract to hepatic vein fistulae occur in the areas of chronic inflammation and fibrosis (5); thus only a proportion of the total liver blood flow actually perfuses hepatic parenchymal cells. A consequence of the distorted vascular bed is to increase hepatic resistance and cause portal vein pressure to rise. Collateral veins outside the liver between the portal and systemic venous circulation dilate and are able to divert up to 60% of blood flow in the splanchnic and mesenteric veins from the liver (6).

Providing that hepatic regeneration compensates for liver cell injury, function will be maintained during the early development of cirrhosis and the patients will be asymptomatic. However as chronic liver disease progresses, regeneration fails to compensate for parenchymal damage and hepatic function becomes compromised. This is reflected by a decreased rate of protein synthesis with a consequent fall in serum albumin and coagulation factors and in a decrease in mixed function oxidase enzyme concentrations in liver tissue (3).

In summary, the cardinal features of chronic cirrhosis vary little with etiology and include a) parenchymal damage of varying degrees, b) grossly distorted architecture in which islands of regenerating tissue develop, c) the development of portal systemic vascular shunts both within the liver and outside it and d) failure of hepatic metabolic function. All of these factors can potentially affect drug metabolism. It is possible that the measurement of kinetic parameters of model drugs might be able to define the underlying pathophysiological state of the patient and allow the prediction of how the disposition of other drugs which are usually eliminated by the liver, might be influenced.

Influence of Chronic Liver Disease on Hepatic Clearance

Dextro-propranolol has been used in a study of the influence of chronic liver disease on drug disposition as a model of a drug which is eliminated by metabolism by the liver (7) with a high intrinsic hepatic clearance (8). It has extensive tissue distribution and has high protein binding (9). The d-isomer of propranolol was chosen for this study, as it is devoid of β-adrenergic blocking properties and therefore does not reduce liver blood flow like the l-isomer of the clinically used racemic mixture (10). Importantly, the disposition of propranolol was compared with that of two other model drugs. Indocyanine green (ICG) is a drug which has a high intrinsic hepatic clearance having hepatic extraction ratios in man which vary from 50-80% (11,12). In contrast to propranolol, ICG is not metabolized but is entirely eliminated by active uptake into hepatic parenchymal cells. It is then transported to bile and once excreted in the small intestine is not reabsorbed (13). These properties make it a suitable indicator for measurement of liver blood flow utilizing the Fick principle with direct measurement of the hepatic extraction ratio. Antipyrine (14) is a drug with a low intrinsic hepatic clearance which is slowly and completely metabolized prior to elimination (15). Because its hepatic clearance is less than 2% of liver blood flow, antipyrine hepatic clearance approximates its intrinsic hepatic clearance and is independent of liver blood flow, reflecting only the activity of the enzymes involved. The kinetics of these three drugs were investigated in each of a carefully selected group of patients with chronic liver disease. Patients with acute, acute on chronic or obstructive liver disease and patients receiving drugs known to be able to induce hepatic microsomal enzyme activity were excluded.

As might have been predicted the clearance of all three drugs was reduced in liver disease. Further, in keeping with earlier data with antipyrine (16,17) the greatest reductions in the clearance were found in patients with low serum albumin concentrations, raised serum bilirubin concentrations and prolonged prothrombin times. There was, however, little or no correlation with other tests of liver function such as SGOT, SGPT and alkaline phosphatase. These correlations are to some extent dependent on patient selection. For instance a raised bilirubin in the absence of acute liver cell damage or biliary obstruction is a poor prognostic sign in chronic liver disease. However a raised serum bilirubin in acute hepatitis is not a discriminating test of function due to the complexity of bilirubin disposition. Similarly, if only patients with acute hepatitis had been selected it is possible that a raised SGPT might have been a better index of the extent of liver damage than the serum albumin. This raises one of the great problems of evaluating drug elimination in hepatic disease: that is the failure to find a precise quantitative estimate of hepatic function. Indeed it has even been suggested that the clearance of a model drug such as antipyrine might be a more rational and quantitative evaluation of the severity of chronic liver disease than the usual routine liver function tests (17).

The explanation for the reduced drug clearance is simplest in the case of antipyrine, as this compound is so poorly extracted that its elimination depends only on enzyme activity (i.e. intrinsic hepatic clearance) which could arise as a result of a defect in either quality or quantity of the enzyme or both. In the case of propranolol and ICG, reductions in both intrinsic hepatic clearance and hepatic blood flow could potentially contribute to reductions in clearance.

An important further observation was a positive correlation between the clearances of antipyrine, d-propranolol and ICG (Fig. 1) despite different modes of drug elimination. This type of observation has also been seen with other groups of compounds including antipyrine and galactose (17) and antipyrine, lidocaine and acetaminophen (18).

In theory, the positive correlation between high and low clearance drugs could arise if flow and intrinsic hepatic clearance falls in parallel. Were this to be the case, the perfusion limited pharmacokinetic model of Rowland et al (1) would suggest that hepatic extraction should remain constant. However direct measurement of the hepatic extraction ratio of several drugs with a high intrinsic hepatic clearance including ICG (11,19,20), bromsulphalein (21,22) and galactose (23) have demonstrated a reduction in hepatic extraction in patients with chronic liver disease (Table I). The reduction in both hepatic clearance and hepatic extraction ratio implies that intrinsic hepatic clearance must fall to a greater extent than liver blood flow. For example, from the mean data presented in Table I, chronic liver disease reduced the liver blood flow by only 15% while the mean reduction in intrinsic hepatic clearance of the various model drugs was reduced by 72%.

There are two possible explanations for the parallel reduction in the clearance of drugs whose elimination is rate limited by either flow or enzyme activity. Firstly, there could be a reduction in the ability of each cell to eliminate drug while blood flow is maintained. This might be called "the sick cell theory". Thus cellular injury would decrease the intrinsic hepatic clearance of both high and low clearance drugs. This would explain the reduction in actual clearance of antipyrine. However in the absence of

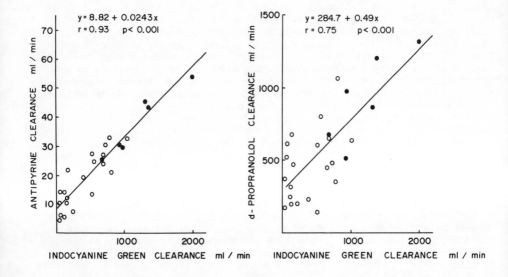

Fig. 1. The relationship between the clearance of indocyanine
green, d-propranolol and antipyrine in 6 normal subjects (●) and 20 patients with chronic liver disease
(○) (adapted from ref. 14 and 9).

significant reduction in flow, decreases in the intrinsic hepatic clearance
of highly extracted compounds should cause a lesser reduction in actual drug
clearance. Therefore, to explain the proportionate fall in clearance of high
and low extraction drugs we must postulate that the intrinsic hepatic clearance of propranolol and ICG is effected more than the intrinsic hepatic clearance of antipyrine. While this is possible, an alternative explanation is
that chronic liver disease is associated with a reduced mass of cells which
function relatively normally and are normally perfused. This might be called
"the intact hepatocyte hypothesis". The reduced extraction of high clearance
drugs would then be due to the presence of intrahepatic shunts which have
been anatomically demonstrated by Popper et al (5). This explanation would
suggest that the major reason for a reduction in drug clearance would be a
reduction in the perfused mass of drug metabolizing enzyme in the liver rather
than a change in Km or amount of enzyme per unit mass of liver. There is
very little evidence of the relationship between 'in vitro' microsomal enzyme
activity and 'in vivo' drug clearance in experimental animal models and even
less in man. However, it is of interest that there was little variation in
concentration of cytochrome P450, and activity of aminopyrine demethylation,
p-nitrosanisole demethylation and NADPH-cytochrome-c-reductase in liver biop-
sy specimens from patients with mild liver disease. These parameters only
decreased in patients with very severely compromised hepatic function (3).

Table I

Author ref.	Marker Drug	Number of Subjects	In Normal Subjects		% Reduction	
			Hepatic Extraction Ratio	Total Clearance	Intrinsic Hepatic Clearance	Estimated L.B.F.
19	ICG	20	.70	641	-50	+6
11	ICG	11	.62	905	-72	-53
23	galactose	24	.88	1460	-72	+4.6
19	BSP	20	.61	685	-55	+7.0
22	BSP	120	.60	920	-83	-25
20	ICG	17	.65	906	-87.5	-7
21	BSP	20	.66	1008		
26	BSP*	10a			-77	-2
		10b			-82	-48
					-72	-15

Examples from the Literature of Direct Measurement of Hepatic Extraction Ratio and Hepatic Clearance Used to Calculate Estimated Total Liver Blood Flow (L.B.F.) Using the Fick Principle. The reduction in estimated intrinsic hepatic clearance and estimated L.B.F. of patients with chronic liver disease has been expressed as a percentage of normal (ICG indocyanine green, BSP bromsulphalein). *A study in patients (a) before and (b) after end-to-side surgical portacaval anastomosis.

Whatever the truth of the matter, and the two hypothesis are not mutually exclusive, the concept that altered drug clearance in chronic liver disease is due largely to a reduction in normally perfused and fully functional liver cell mass has a certain practical appeal, in that it allows a quantitative comparison with the normal situation and suggests that information with a model drug, such as antipyrine may be extrapolated to several other drugs even though they are handled very differently. In addition it serves to emphasize the functional importance of actual organ clearance.

Protein Binding in Liver Disease

As chronic liver disease progresses, hepatic synthetic function deteriorates; this is reflected by a decrease in the production of plasma proteins particularly in the synthesis of albumin (see Chapter 7, Table II). In such patients the extensive protein binding of propranolol is impaired (9). A reduction from 87.8 ± 5.6% binding in normal subjects to 82.3 ± 5.7% in patients with chronic liver disease represents a 45% increase in unbound fraction of drug. Propranolol not only binds to albumin, but also binds to other plasma proteins. Thus, it is not surprising that changes in binding do not correlate with changes in serum albumin. This is in contrast to amobarbital, where changes in protein binding are dependent on changes in the serum albumin (24). (See Table IV of Chapter 4) The explanation of intersubject variation in propranolol binding remains unknown. The relationship between protein binding and the apparent volume of distribution is consistent with the physiological approach to distribution developed by Gillette (25), with a linear relationship between the fraction of unbound drug and the apparent volume of distribution in normal subjects and patients with cirrhosis without fluid retention (Fig. 2). It is noteworthy that small changes in protein binding have a considerable influence on drug distribution, emphasizing that protein binding helps to retain drug in the vascular compartment making less drug available for tissue distribution.

A further factor influencing distribution is the total size of the plasma protein pool. The development of ascites is associated with a two fold increases in the volume of distribution of propranolol in patients with a similar degree of protein binding (Fig. 2). Using the volume of distribution of indocyanine green as a measure of plasma volume, if it is assumed that protein concentrations in ascites and plasma are similar and that the free drug to tissue ratio remains constant, then the increase in extravascular volume in those patients with clinical ascites could be estimated to be approximately 5 L.

The Influences of Portacaval Anastomosis

With the development of portal hypertension, a porta-systemic collateral circulation opens between gastric and esophageal veins just below the mucosal surface. These vessels are at risk of rupturing and causing massive hemorrhage. In patients who have had a hemorrhage, the risk of future hemorrhage can be reduced by surgical diversion of portal vein blood from the liver to the inferior vena cava. This would be expected to reduce total liver flow and therefore the clearance of drugs with a high intrinsic hepatic clearance. However, intrinsic hepatic clearance decreases with the progression of chronic liver disease, and this rate of reduction of hepatic function may be

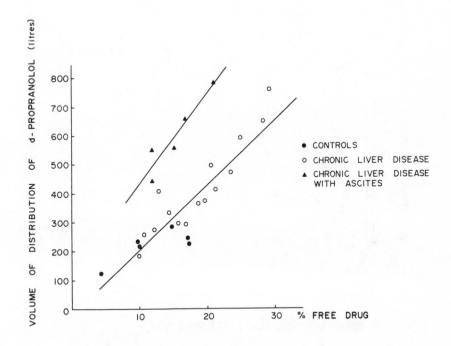

Fig. 2.   The relationship between percentage unbound propranolol
and volume of distribution in normal subjects (●) patients with chronic liver disease without ascites (o)
and patients with chronic liver disease with ascites
(▲) (from ref. 9).

increased by the surgical operation. Thus, changes in clearance due to
changes in flow need to be evaluated in patients with comparable function.
Fortunately antipyrine clearance offers a quantitative measure of drug metabolizing activity which is independent of flow. A comparison of the relationship of the clearance of ICG and antipyrine in patients with or without
such surgery demonstrates that surgical venous diversion reduces ICG clearance by approximately 300 ml/min (Fig. 3) which is similar to the reduction
in flow measured by the Fick principle before and after surgery (26). It is
of interest to note, that the mean estimated intrinsic hepatic clearance of
this group of patients had decreased postoperatively (Table I).

A further implication of diversion of blood from liver to systemic circulation is that drug administered orally will pass directly into the systemic circulation, preventing a first-pass effect reducing the drugs bioavailability. This has been confirmed in a single patient with propranolol (27)

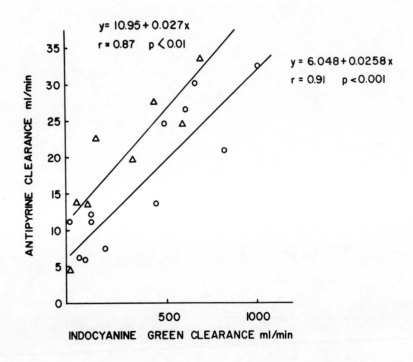

Fig. 3. The relationship between the clearance of antipyrine
         compared to the clearance of indocyanine green. (○)
         patients with chronic liver disease without a surgical
         portacaval anastomosis. (△) patients with chronic
         liver disease and a surgical portacaval anastomosis.
         Both correlations were significant (p<0.05). The
         linear regression lines are parallel with significantly
         different y intercepts (from ref. 14).

and in the dog (28) and implies that oral administration of high clearance
drugs with a low therapeutic ratio could be hazardous in such patients.

Summary

    Although there are many different causes for chronic liver disease, the
final pathological consequences tend to be similar. Cell injury, an inflammatory response and active regeneration of hepatocytes all contribute to
cause a distortion of the normal hepatic architecture and vascular bed. In
addition, when hepatic regeneration fails to compensate for liver damage,

there is a failure in hepatic function. These underlying pathophysiological changes have the potential of influencing normal drug disposition in many different but explicable ways.

There is an increasing body of data confirming that the disposition of many drugs is altered in chronic liver disease. However, until recently the mechanism of the alteration has remained uncertain. The development of a physiological approach to understanding the physiology of drug disposition has allowed a critical evaluation of the relative influence of changes in hepatic drug eliminating activity, liver blood flow, protein binding and the architecture of blood supply to the liver on the kinetics of three model drugs, namely d-propranolol, indocyanine green and antipyrine. The changes observed suggest that,firstly, knowledge of the kinetics of a model drug can provide a quantitative assessment of specific aspects of hepatic function which might be of value in the assessment of the underlying disease process. Secondly, that it might be possible to use a model drug to predict optimal therapeutic regimes thereby rationalizing drug therapy in patients with chronic liver disease.

References

1. M. Rowland, L. Z. Benet and G. G. Graham. Clearance concepts in pharmacokinetics. J. Pharmacokin. Biopharm. 1:123-136 (1973).
2. G. R. Wilkinson and D. G. Shand. A physiological approach to hepatic drug clearance. Clin. Pharm. Ther. 18:377-390 (1975).
3. G. Schoene, R. A. Fleischmann, H. Remmer and H. F. Oldershausen. Determination of drug metabolizing enzymes in needle biopsies of human liver. Europ. J. Clin. Pharm. 4:65-73 (1972).
4. B. May, D. Helmstaedt, L. Bustgens and A. McLean. A relation between cytochrome P450 in liver biopsies and drug metabolism in patients with liver disease and in morphine addiction. Clin. Sci. 46:11P (1974).
5. H. Popper, H. Elias and D. E. Petty. Vascular pattern of the cirrhotic liver. Am. J. Clin. Path. 22:717-729 (1954).
6. R. Groszmann, B. Kotelanski, J. N. Cohn and I. M. Khatri. Quantitation of portasystemic shunting from the splenic and mesenteric beds in alcoholic liver disease. Am. J. Med. 53:715-722 (1972).
7. P. A. Bond. Metabolism of propranolol (Inderal); a potent, specific β-adrenergic receptor blocking agent. Nature 213:721-723 (1967).
8. G. H. Evans, A. S. Nies and D. G. Shand. The disposition of propranolol, III. Decreased half-life and volume of distribution as a result of plasma binding in man, monkey, dog and rat. J. Pharm. Exp. Ther. 186:114-122 (1973).
9. R. A. Branch, J. James and A. E. Read. A study of factors influencing drug disposition in chronic liver disease using the model drug (+)-propranolol. Brit. J. Clin. Pharm. 3:243-249 (1976).
10. A. S. Nies, G. H. Evans and D. G. Shand. Regional hemodynamic effects of beta-adrenergic blockade with propranolol in the unanesthetized primate. Am. Ht. J. 85:97-102 (1973).
11. J. Caesar, S. Shaldon, L. Chiandussi, L. Guevara and S. Sherlock. The use of indocyanine green in the measurement of hepatic blood flow and as a test of hepatic function. Clin. Sci. 21:43-57 (1961).

12. G. R. Cherrick, S. W. Stein, C. M. Leevy and C. S. Davidson. Indo-cyanine green: Observations on its physical properties, plasma decay and hepatic extraction. J. Clin. Invest. 39:592-600 (1960).

13. H. O. Wheeler, W. I. Cranston and J. I. Meltzer. Hepatic uptake and biliary excretion of indocyanine green in the dog. Proc. Soc. Exp. Biol. (New York) 99:11-16 (1958).

14. R. A. Branch, J. A. James and A. E. Read. The clearance of antipyrine and indocyanine green in normal subjects and in patients with chronic liver disease. Clin. Pharm. Ther. 20: 81-89 (1976).

15. B. B. Brodie and J. Axelrod. Fate of antipyrine in man. J. Pharm. Ther. 98:97-104 (1950).

16. R. A. Branch, C. M. Herbert and A. E. Read. Determinants of serum anti-pyrine half-lives in patients with liver disease. Gut 14:569-573 (1973).

17. P. B. Andreason, L. Ranek, B. E. Statland and N. Tygstrup. Clearance of antipyrine-dependence of quantitative liver function. Europ. J. Clin. Invest. 4:129-134 (1974).

18. J. A. H. Forrest, N. D. C. Finlayson, K. K. Adjepon-Yomoah and L. F. Prescott. Antipyrine, lignocaine and paracetamol metabolism in chronic liver disease. Gut 67:790 (1974).

19. C. M. Leevy, C. L. Mendenhall, W. Lesko and M. M. Howard. Estimation of hepatic blood flow with indocyanine green. J. Clin. Invest. 41:1169-1179 (1962).

20. J. N. Cohn, I. M. Khatri, R. J. Groszmann and B. Kotelanski. Hepatic blood flow in alcoholic liver disease measured by an indicator dilution technique. Am. J. Med. 53:704-714 (1972).

21. W. E. Bradley, F. J. Ingelfinger, G. P. Bradley and J. J. Curry. The estimation of hepatic blood flow in man. J. Clin. Invest. 24:890-897 (1945).

22. S. E. Bradley, F. J. Ingelfinger and G. P. Bradley. Hepatic circulation in cirrhosis of the liver. Circ. 5:419-429 (1952).

23. N. Tygstrup and K. Winker. Galactose blood clearance as a measure of hepatic blood flow. Clin. Sci. 17:1-9 (1958).

24. G. E. Mawer, N. E. Miller and L. A. Turnburg. Metabolism of amylobarbi-tone in patients with chronic liver disease. Brit. J. Pharm. 44:549-560 (1972).

25. J. R. Gillette. Factors affecting drug metabolism. Annals of New York Academy of Science 179:43-66 (1971).

26. A. G. Redeker, H. M. Geller and T. B. Reynolds. Hepatic wedge pressure, blood flow, vascular resistance and oxygen consumption in cirrhosis be-fore and after end-to side portacaval shunt. J. Clin. Invest. 37:606-618 (1958).

27. D. G. Shand and R. E. Rangno. The disposition of propranolol I. Elim-ination during oral absorption in man. Pharm. 7:159-168 (1972).

28. R. Gugler, P. Lain and D. L. Azarnoff. Effect of portacaval shunt on the disposition of drugs with and without first pass effect. J. Pharm. Exp. Ther. 195:416-423 (1975).

Chapter 6

PHARMACOKINETIC IMPLICATIONS OF CHRONIC DRUG

TREATMENT IN EPILEPSY: CARBAMAZEPINE

Rene' H. Levy, William H. Pitlick,
Allan S. Troupin & John R. Green (deceased)

Epilepsy is a group of related disorders arising from excessive
neuronal discharges within the brain. The common feature of all forms
of epilepsy is the recurring nature of the disturbances. The experience
accumulated to date indicates that although the psychological and social
aspects of treatment bear much significance, pharmacotherapeutic agents
remain the primary tools in the control of epilepsy. Treatment is aimed
at preventing the recurrence of the symptoms and is thus of a chronic
nature.

In epilepsy, effects of the disease state on the pharmacokinetics
are not mediated through pathological changes associated with the clinical state of the patient (changes in body hemodynamics or in renal function). Nevertheless, the epileptic patient presents several challenges
to the pharmacokineticist:

a) drug treatment is of a chronic nature;

b) drug withdrawal can be associated with severe clinical
    consequences;

c) a significant proportion of antiepileptic drugs are enzyme
    inducers and

d) polypharmacy is generally the rule.

As a result of a) and b) above, classical single dose pharmacokinetic studies become difficult, if not impossible. As a result of
c) and d) above, inter-patient variability in pharmacokinetic parameters
(such as clearance and biological half life) is so large that it almost
negates their usefulness in the therapeutic management of patients.

These problems are magnified in the case of new drugs as was our
experience with carbamazepine (Tegretol[R]). Reported values for its
biological half life ranged from 8 to 55 hrs and consequently, recommended dosing frequencies ranged from q.d (once a day) to t.i.d. (three
times a day). Thus, as far as providing any assistance in rational
therapeutic management with carbamazepine, the promise of pharmacokinetics was not realized. The studies to be described were undertaken in

an attempt to elucidate this situation.

Half Life Values of Carbamazepine in Patients

In a pilot study designed to compare the efficacy of carbamazepine to that of diphenylhydantoin, Troupin et al. (1) measured the half life of carbamazepine in eight patients following a four-month treatment period with the drug. They found values ranging between 8.5 and 19.0 hrs with a mean of 12.1 $\pm$ 3.2 hrs.

Single Dose Studies[1]

Single dose studies were then undertaken in a group of 6 normal human volunteers (mean age 25.8 $\pm$ 3.8 yr and mean weight 69.3 $\pm$ 18.8 kg). Five treatments were administered to the subjects according to a randomized crossover design: 3 mg/kg (treatment D), 6 mg/kg (treatment A), and 9 mg/kg (treatment E) of carbamazepine in a propylene glycol solution; 6 mg/kg as a commercial tablet (treatment B), and 6 mg/kg as the same tablet with meal (treatment C).

Carbamazepine was relatively rapidly absorbed from the propylene glycol solution with a mean peak concentration (C_{max}) of 6.46 $\pm$ 0.88 μg/ml and an average time to achieve maximum serum concentration (T_{max}) of 3.20 $\pm$ 1.30 hr (Table I). Both extent and rate of absorption were significantly reduced for the tablet dosage form (empty stomach).

Table I. Pharmacokinetic Parameters of Carbamazepine from a Single Dose Study in a Group of Six Normal Human Volunteers

Parameter	Tablet (6 mg/Kg)	Solution (3 mg/Kg)	Solution (6 mg/Kg)	Solution (9 mg/Kg)	Tablet with Meal (6 mg/Kg)
C_{max} (μg/ml)	4.52[a] 0.80[b]	3.87 1.20	6.46 0.88	8.78 1.89	5.68 0.21
T_{max} (hr)	7.17 3.71	3.80 4.5	3.20 1.30	3.85 1.62	7.00 2.00
$T_{1/2}$ (hr)	35.3 10.0	32.6 6.8	30.6 4.6	32.6 12.3	33.1 9.2

[a]Mean   [b]Standard Deviation

[1]A full report of these studies has been published. (2)

The bioavailability of the tablet compared to the solution was 79% (p = 0.015) and ranged between 56% and 109%. Also, T_{max}, 7.17 ± 3.7 hr, was significantly prolonged (p = 0.02) and the maximum concentration for the tablet (4.52 ± 0.8 μg/ml) was significantly lower than for the solution (p = 0.001). Giving the tablet with a meal (treatment C) increased the bioavailability, but this difference was not significant (p = 0.076). The peak concentration, 5.68 ± 0.21 μg/ml, however was greater (p = 0.003) with no change in T_{max} (Table I).

The range of individual elimination half-lives ($T_{1/2}$) for treatments A, B and C was 21.2 to 52.9 hr. The corresponding mean half-lives were 30.6 ± 4.6, 35.3 ± 10.0, and 33.1 ± 9.2 hr, respectively (no significant differences between treatments). The fraction of dose excreted unchanged in 72 hr was less than 1% for these three treatments, indicating that the drug is essentially completely metabolized.

There was a linear relationship between C_{max} and dose in the 3-9 mg/kg range (Table I). There was no significant change in T_{max} or absorption half-life for the 3 doses. At 3, 6 and 9 mg/kg, the elimination half-life was 32.6 ± 6.8, 30.6 ± 4.6, and 32.6 ± 12.3 hr, respectively (no significant difference in half-life for the 3 doses). There was no change in the fraction of dose excreted unchanged in the dosage range studied (less than 1% of the dose for the three doses).

Chronic Dosing Studies in Normal Human Volunteers

In view of the difference in half life values found in volunteers and in patients, the following study was undertaken to find out whether carbamazepine given chronically alone to normal human volunteers is able to affect its own elimination half-life.

Six normal drug-free volunteers (mean age 25.5 ± 6.4 years, mean weight 60.8 ± 20.1 kg) participated in this study (subjects different from the previous single dose study). A control single dose study was first initiated where each subject received a 6 mg/kg dose. One week later, all six subjects received 6 mg/kg as a tablet once daily in the morning for 22 days.

In the single dose study, sixteen blood samples of 10 ml of blood each were collected (by venipuncture and heparin lock) over a 72 hr period. During the multiple dose study, seven blood samples of 10 ml each were collected over a 24 hr period on days 8, 15, and 22. In addition, 48 and 72 hr samples were collected following administration of the last dose on day 22. Urine was collected for a 72 hr period in the single dose study and 24 hr urine collections were made on days 8, 15, and 22 of the chronic dosing study.

Serum and urine samples were analyzed for unchanged carbamazepine by gas-liquid chromatography as described previously (2).

The data from this study was tested for significant differences by pairwise comparisons using the SPSS program T-TEST.

1. Single Dose Studies

The mean C_{max} for the six subjects receiving a single dose of
6 mg/kg was 5.47 + 1.19 µg/ml. The average T_{max} observed experimentally
was 7.50 + 2.5 hrs. The mean $T_{1/2}$ for these six subjects following
a single dose was 33.89 + 3.51 hours. Less than 1% of the dose was
excreted unchanged in the urine. These values are in very close agreement with the values previously obtained in the bioavailability and
dose-dependency studies (Table I).

2. Multiple Dose Studies

a) Experimental Data: The observed values for C_{min} (concentration
at end of dosing interval), C_{max} and total body clearance (CL_T) were
compared to the values predicted using single dose parameters. The C_{max}
values of 9.63, 8.38 and 8.40 µg/ml at the end of the first, second and
third week were significantly less than the predicted value of 13.58
µg/ml (p = .0015). The mean C_{min} values of 5.62, 4.28 and 3.83 µg/ml
at the end of the first, second and third week were also significantly
less than the predicted value of 9.88 µg/ml (p < .0005). The mean $T_{1/2}$
was also reduced from 33.89 hrs to 19.82 hrs (Fig. 1).

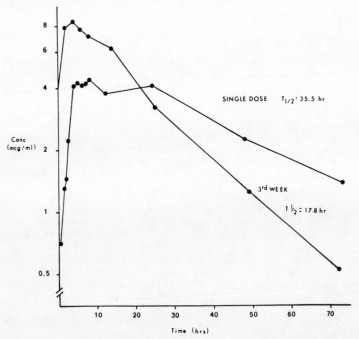

Fig. 1. Serum concentration-time curves for the single dose
study and days 22-25 of the chronic dosing study
illustrating the change in biological half-life
(Subject DM).

90

The mean CL_T increased significantly from .0207 L/Kg/hr to .0344 L/Kg/hr at day 8 and continued to increase at days 15 and 22 (p < .0005) (Figs. 2 and 3).

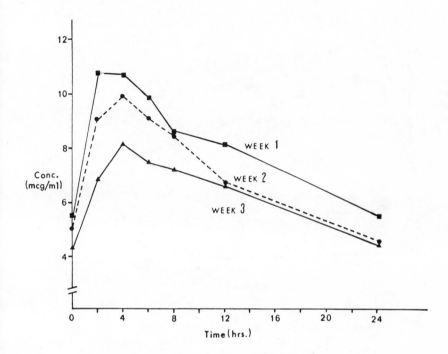

Fig. 2. Steady state serum concentrations for days 8, 15 and 22 during chronic dosing illustrating the decrease in C_{max} and C_{min} (Subject EL).

Less than 1% of the drug was excreted unchanged during any 24 hr dosage interval. It is worthwhile to note that C_{max} and C_{min} continued to change between the first and third week of treatment. Significant reductions (p < .05) were seen in C_{max} and C_{min} between days 8 and 22 (Figs. 2 and 3). C_{max} and C_{min} decreased from 9.6 μg/ml and 5.6 μg/ml respectively at the end of the first week to 8.4 μg/ml and 3.8 μg/ml respectively at the end of the third week.

b) Biochemical and Pharmacokinetic Interpretations: The decreases in steady state serum concentrations and in elimination half-life during chronic dosing are probably related to auto-induction. Such an effect has been documented for carbamazepine in rats (3). In addition, carbamazepine has been shown to reduce the half-lives of several other drugs (4-6). Furthermore, studies in our laboratories have shown that steady state levels of carbamazepine decrease exponentially during a one week infusion in rhesus monkeys (7).

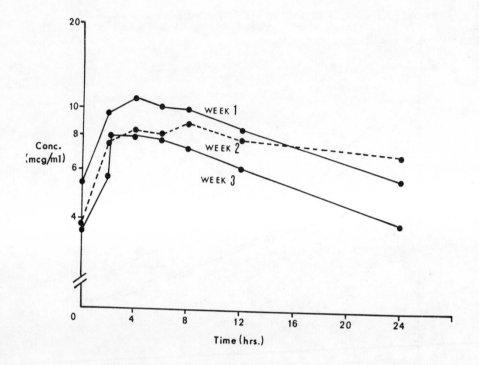

Fig. 3. Steady state serum concentrations for days 8, 15 and 22 during chronic dosing illustrating the decrease in C_{max} and C_{min} (Subject RO).

A pharmacokinetic model with an exponentially increasing elimination rate constant $K_E(t)$ has been recently described to account for the exponential auto-induction phenomenon (8):

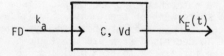

In this model, $K_E(t)$ is given by:

$$K_E(t) = K_E^\infty - (K_E^\infty - K_E^0)e^{-K_I t} \qquad \text{(Eq. 1)}$$

92

where C is the concentration at any time in the one compartment of volume Vd; K_E^0 and K_E^∞ represent the elimination rate constants obtained from single dose and chronic dosing studies, respectively; K_I represents a first order <u>induction</u> rate constant; FD is the fraction of dose D absorbed; and $\overline{k_a}$ a first order absorption rate constant.

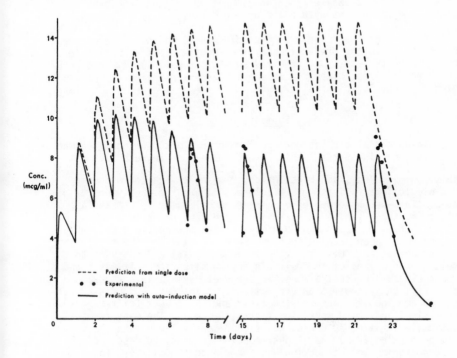

Fig. 4. Comparison of serum concentrations observed for days 8, 15, and 22 with single dose predictions and those based on the auto-induction model (Subject JH).

The data shown in Fig. 4 suggest that there is a good agreement between experimental values and predictions of the auto-induction model. The induction half-lives obtained in six subjects ranged from 2.2 to 6.4 days with a mean of 4.0 ± 1.6 days.

Conclusions

These studies suggest that the spread in biological half lives reported for carbamazepine is probably linked to the phenomenon of auto-induction. Single dose studies consistently yield half lives around thirty hours while chronic dosing studies yield values generally less than twenty hours. It is likely that the short half lives encountered in epileptic patients are due to auto-induction during chronic dosing. It is also possible that the phenomenon of auto-induction is dose dependent in humans.[2] In that case, the extent of auto-induction seen in patients would be larger than that observed at the low doses used in normal human volunteers and would yield biological half lives even shorter than those observed in the present study. Furthermore, an additional enzyme inducing effect brought about by concurrent medication (phenytoin and/or phenobarbital) is also possible.

It is apparent that single dose studies in normal human volunteers are not relevant to the predictions of therapeutic needs of epileptic patients. Nevertheless, such single dose studies were useful in generating "control" pharmacokinetic parameters, thereby enabling an understanding of a complex clinical picture.

Summary

Single-dose oral studies were performed in a group of normal human volunteers receiving 5 treatments of carbamazepine (Tegretol[R]): A (solution, 6 mg/Kg); B (tablet, 6 mg/Kg); C (tablet with meal, 6 mg/Kg); D (solution, 3 mg/Kg), and E (solution, 9 mg/Kg). The corresponding mean biological half-lives were 31, 35 and 33 hrs for treatments C, D and E. In a second group of drug-free normal human volunteers a single dose study (tablet, 6 mg/Kg) was conducted prior to a multiple dose study (tablet, 6 mg/Kg once a day for 22 consecutive days). A one compartment open model with first order elimination (Model I) was found adequate to describe the single dose data and was used to formulate predictions of the multiple dosing situation. It was found that experimental concentrations (measured at days 7, 15 and 22-25) were significantly lower than predictions. Also, C_{max} and C_{min} decreased continuously between the first and third week (differences between first and third week significant, ($p < .05$). The mean terminal biological half-life, 19.8 hrs, was significantly lower than the single dose value ($p < .05$). A pharmacokinetic model to describe the phenomenon of self-induction was formulated (Model II). There was good agreement between experimental findings and the predictions of Model II.

---

[2]Studies in our laboratory show that it is in fact the case for carbamazepine in rhesus monkeys (unpublished data).

94

Acknowledgments

This study was supported by a grant from Ciba Geigy Corporation and in part by NIH contract NO1-NS-0-2281 and a Grant NS04053 awarded by National Institute of Neurological and Communicative Disorders and Stroke, PHS/DHEW.

A portion of this research was done at the Clinical Research Center at the University of Washington and was supported by NIH (Grant RR-37).

The technical assistance of John Neal was greatly appreciated.

References

1. A. S. Troupin, J. R. Green, and R. H. Levy. Carbamazepine as an anticonvulsant: A pilot study. Neurology. 24:863-869 (1974).

2. R. H. Levy, W. H. Pitlick, A. S. Troupin, J. R. Green, and J. M. Neal. Pharmacokinetics of carbamazepine in normal man. Clin. Pharmacol. Ther. 17:657-668 (1975).

3. P. L. Morselli, P. Biandrate, A. Frigerio, and S. Garattini. Pharmacokinetics of carbamazepine in rats and humans. Eur. J. Clin. Invest. 2:297 (1972).

4. O. Penttila, P. J. Neuvonen, K. Aho, and R. Lehtovaara. Interaction between doxycycline and some antiepileptic drugs. Brit. Med. J. 2:470-472 (1974).

5. J. M. Hansen, K. Siersbaek-Nielsen, and L. Skovsted. Carbamazepine induced acceleration of diphenylhydantoin and warfarin metabolism in man. Clin. Pharmacol. Ther. 12:539-543 (1971).

6. R. Ronfeld and L. Z. Benet. Carbamazepine induced changes in the pharmacokinetics of diphenylhydantoin and carbamazepine. In Abstracts of the 121st Annual Meeting of the APhA Academy of Pharmaceutical Sciences, Chicago, Vol. 4, Washington, D.C., 1974, p. 119.

7. W. H. Pitlick and R. H. Levy. A pharmacokinetic model with capacity-limited elimination following zero-order infusion. In Abstracts of the 19th National Meeting of the APhA Academy of Pharmaceutical Sciences, Atlanta, Vol. 5, Washington, D.C., 1975, p. 121.

8. W. H. Pitlick, R. H. Levy, A. S. Troupin, and J. R. Green. A pharmacokinetic model to describe self-induced decreases in steady state concentration of carbamazepine. J. Pharm. Sci. 65:462-463 (1976).

III. PROTEIN BINDING

Chapter 7

PHARMACOKINETICS IN DISEASE STATES CHANGING PROTEIN BINDING

William J. Jusko

The pervasive nature of drug-protein binding has attracted considerable attention in pharmacology and pharmacokinetics. This has occurred because of both the ease of carrying out *in vitro* binding measurements and the recognition or presumption of the role of binding in determining drug effects and disposition.

This report will focus on three areas in relation to the effects of disease in drug binding and pharmacokinetics: examination of the materials in the human body which are capable of binding drugs, consideration of the alteration of proteins and the degree of drug-protein binding in various diseases, and an overview of the role of protein binding in determining the pharmacokinetics and pharmacologic effects of some specific drugs.

Drug Binding Components

Albumin Distribution

The major plasma and tissue protein which is usually responsible for the non-specific binding of most drugs is albumin. Studies of the dynamics of albumin have usually involved the intravenous injection of I^{131} or I^{125}-labeled albumin (1). In spite of its large molecular weight (69,000), albumin is not exclusively retained in the plasma but is also distributed extravascularly. The extravascular space consists of many different anatomical compartments, each of which has its own characteristic pool size and exchange rate with the vascular compartment. Most plasma disappearance curves of labeled albumin can be resolved into three components. The component with the largest half-life of about 17-18 days essentially reflects the catabolic rate of albumin. The other two components with half-lives of about 6 hours and about 28 hours indicate that there are at least two distinct groups of extravascular compartments which contain albumin and are in equilibrium with the vascular compartment. The model most often used to depict albumin distribution is a three compartment model with an intra-vascular (plasma) compartment and two extravascular compartments. In those tissues with discontinuous capillaries (such as the liver, spleen, and intestine) and high plasma perfusion rates, distribution occurs rapidly and is represented by the extravascular compartment with the smaller volume of distribution. Those tissues with continuous capillaries (such as the muscle and skin) and with small plasma perfusion rates are represented by the larger and more slowly exchanging extravascular compartment (1-3).

The largest fraction of extravascular albumin is located in the skin which contains approximately 18% of the total exchangeable albumin. This high albumin content of the skin is related to the large volume of extra-cellular fluid in this tissue, namely about 60% of skin weight. Similarly, the large mass (40-45% body weight) of muscle accounts for the fact that it contains about 15% of total exchangeable albumin (2).

Figure 1 shows the relationship between the normalized intravascular and extravascular masses of albumin. The data were obtained from several different literature sources and represent a total of 83 patients (3). The data in the graph fall approximately in the shape of an elongated ellipse with the greatest density of points located toward the center of the ellipse. At this point values of 2.24 gm/kg and 1.57 gm/kg for the extravascular (EV) and intravascular (IV) masses, respectively, reflect the highest probability of occurrence of the mean ratio. The average EV/IV ratio is 1.43 indicating that 59% of the total exchangeable albumin is located in the extravascular compartment. The great degree of scatter in the data shown in Figure 1 also indicates that patients differ considerably in distribution of albumin and that measurements of plasma protein concentrations may not be a consistent index of total body stores of the protein.

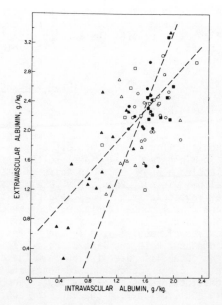

Fig. 1. Relationship between extra-vascular and intravascular albumin contents in 83 patients. Data were gathered from 6 sources by Jusko and Gretch (3).

Factors Affecting the Albumin Content of Body Compartments

Many pathophysiological states will cause a change (mostly lowering) of plasma albumin concentrations as a result of modifications in the synthesis rate, catabolic rate, or the distribution between the extravascular and intravascular spaces. Some of the factors that decrease plasma albumin concentrations are summarized in Table I. The extent to which lowered albumin levels occur in various disease states is found in a recent report by Casey (4). About 18% of more than 23,000 patients admitted to one hospital had low serum albumin concentrations.

Table I. Diseases Lowering Plasma Albumin

Small Change		Larger Change
Bone Fractures	Neoplastic Disease	Liver Disease
Freezing	GI Disease	Renal Disease
Myocardial Infarction	Chronic Bronchitis	Burns
Surgery	Cystic Fibrosis	
Acute Infection	Bedrest	
Pregnancy	Smoking	
	Aging	

In acute injury or disease, reduced plasma levels of albumin and increased γ-globulin levels in plasma are thought to be the normal host reaction to injury or infection rather than being a response to any specific disease. Burns, freezing, bone fractures, myocardial infarction, and surgery are followed by decreased plasma albumin levels. Acute febrile infections such as pneumonia, tonsillitis, scarlet fever, rheumatic fever, and peritonitis also cause a decrease in albumin levels and an elevation in γ-globulin levels. Casey (4) reported significant decreases in albumin and increases in globulin concentrations in 17 types of febrile illnesses associated with infections by virus or bacteria which involved 7% of his patients.

Prolonged bedrest or immobilization produces a profound effect on albumin distribution. Five paraplegic patients who were confined to bed for at least two months following an operation showed EV/IV ratios which averaged more than twice the normal value (5).

Surgical procedures can produce a prolonged negative protein balance, largely owing to loss of proteins into the traumetized area and the increased protein demands of the regenerating tissues. For example, abdominal operations cause a decrease in plasma albumin by more than 0.5 gm/dl in about 70% of patients (6).

Burns cause the most pronounced decrease in plasma albumin (7). This occurs, firstly, because the skin contains the largest fraction of extra-vascular albumin and destruction of an appreciable portion of skin results in a significant loss of interstitial albumin. Secondly, capillary permeability is increased after extensive burns and this increased permeability causes albumin depletion from the plasma compartment and marked extravascular pooling of albumin, especially in the initial phase of the burn.

Pregnancy can decrease plasma albumin. Similar, but less pronounced, changes were noted in women receiving oral contraceptives (estrogen/progesterone combinations) (8).

Neoplastic diseases are associated with lower serum albumin. Mider (9) observed that the plasma albumin concentration varies inversely with the stage of the malignant process. As the disease becomes more disseminated, the albumin concentration progressively decreases. Steinfeld (10), in following 83 cancer patients over a period of 1 month to five years, found that serum albumin concentrations fell an average of 1 gm/dl. It appears that both total exchangeable albumin and the intravascular albumin mass are uniformly subnormal in cancer patients due to diminished albumin synthesis.

Liver diseases are the most complex and prevalent of the chronic disorders afflicting man. The liver synthesizes most plasma proteins and hepatic impairment, especially chronic disease, can result in diminished protein levels in the body. A summary of average serum albumin concentrations in various types of hepatic disorders is shown in Table II. Acute toxic hepatitis, hepatic tumors, and various cirrhotic diseases were found to cause the most pronounced decrease in serum albumin levels (11).

Table II. Serum Proteins In Liver Diseases

Disease	Serum Albumin No.	g./L,
Normal	30	38.4
Acute Viral Hepatitis	20	32.9
Acute Toxic Hepatitis	6	25.5
Active Chronic Hepatitis	29	28.7
Chronic Persistant Hepatitis	11	35.6
Cryptogenic Cirrhosis	23	27.3
Primary Biliary Cirrhosis	19	30.9
Alcoholic Cirrhosis	17	30.4
Steatosis	9	37.9
Hepatic Tumors	10	25.7

From Skrede et al. (11)

Neither the kidney nor the gastrointestinal tract play a significant role in albumin disposition in healthy subjects. However, marked elimination of albumin occurs in some diseases affecting these organs. Where the glomeruli and tubules are both affected in chronic renal disease, excessive protein filtration may lead to increased loss of albumin from the body. Nephrosis, in particular, is associated with severe hypoalbuminemia. In one study involving 30 nephrotoxic patients, serum albumin levels were below 1 gm/dl in 6 patients, between 1 and 2 gm/dl in 18 patients, and 6 patients had values in the range of 2.2 to 3.4 gm/dl (12). Nephrosis causes both an increase in the degradation of albumin and a decrease in the intravascular and total exchangeable mass of albumin.

Diseases of all segments of the gastrointestinal tract may diminish plasma albumin. However, protein-losing enteropathy occurs primarily in relationship to two specific processes. Blockage of lymphatics leads to loss of lymph into the gastrointestinal tract. Also, mucosal disease with weeping or direct loss of serum into the gut is seen in inflammatory bowel disorders. In addition, specific conditions such as gastric polyps may cause a large exudation of albumin into the gastrointestinal tract. Hypoalbuminemia is a common finding in patients with disorders complicated by bacterial overgrowth in the intestine which diminish the transport of amino acids across the intestinal membrane (13).

Normal human bronchial secretions contain albumin. In patients with
chronic bronchitis, the albumin loss through the sputum is increased.
Reductions in half-life, extravascular and intravascular mass, total
exchangeable mass, and intravascular concentration of albumin have been
demonstrated in patients with chronic bronchitis (14).

Hypoalbuminemia in cystic fibrosis is usually caused by dilution of the
normal circulating albumin mass in an enlarged plasma volume. In 16 cystic
fibrosis subjects, ten patients had albumin levels less than 3.5 gm/dl while
6 had normal serum levels. The plasma volume of the hypoalbuminemic group
was markedly higher (56.4 ml/kg) than those who had normal albumin values
(43.6 ml/kg). Both total intravascular albumin and EV/IV ratios were in the
normal range for all patients (15).

Control over the upper limits of plasma albumin mass and concentration
is much more effective than that for the lower limits. This, in part,
explains why relatively few disease states are associated with elevated
plasma albumin. Casey (16) reported several disease syndromes which are
associated with elevated serum albumin levels, some of which are listed in
Table III. Ecanow et al. (17) confirmed the findings of Casey in reporting
elevated serum albumin concentrations in 76% of their patients exhibiting
anxiety or agitation.

Table III. Diseases Increasing Plasma Albumin

Neuroses
Psychoses
Schizophrenia
Paranoia
Gynecologic Disorder
Myalgia
Benign Tumor

From Casey et al. (16)

Tissue Binding of Various Drugs

Binding of drugs to plasma proteins has been extensively studied
primarily because the plasma is readily accessible to sampling, can be easily
separated into its constituent macromolecules, and drug-protein interactions
are easily quantitated. Tissue binding studies have none of these advantages
and, as a result, knowledge of the qualitative and quantitative aspects of
the binding of drugs to tissue components is poorly understood. The previous
section showed that albumin, with its extensive distribution into
interstitial fluids, may be the principal drug binding protein in tissues.
However, a number of other binding materials have been found to account for
interaction with some drugs. Some of these are summarized in Table IV.

Table IV. Tissue Binding Of Drugs

Material	Drug Bound
Ligandin	- Various drugs
DNA	- Antineoplastic agents
	- Antimalarial drugs
Melanin	- Psoralins
Calcified Tissues	- Tetracyclines
Mucopolysaccharides	- Amines
Cell Fractions	- Basic lipophilic drugs
Transcortin	- Corticosteroids
Enzymes:	
NA/K T-ATP'ase	- Cardiac glycosides
Dihydrofolate R'ase	- Methotrexate

A major discovery of an important anion binding protein in tissues occurred in the identification of ligandin (18). This protein has a molecular weight of about 42,000 and constitutes about 4 percent of the total cell sap protein of rat liver. Appreciable ligandin concentrations are also found in the tubule cells of kidney and mucosal cells of the small intestine. It has not been detected in plasma, bile, brain, and other tissues. Ligandin binds a number of endogenous and exogenous substances strongly but noncovalently. These compounds include azo dyes, corticosteroids, bilirubin, bromosulphthalein (BSP), carcinogens, and folate (18,19). There is a direct relationship between the hepatic concentration of ligandin and the net flux of bilirubin, BSP, and other organic anions between plasma and the liver cell. Ligandin is a major determinant of selective hepatic uptake of certain small molecules and may also influence the flux of metabolites from the liver into the plasma or bile. The rapidity of hepatic distribution of chemicals with the assistance of ligandin is demonstrated by the uptake of over 50 percent of an intravenous dose of bilirubin within five minutes of injection into a rat (20).

Many drugs, including various antineoplastic compounds, bind to DNA (21). A photosensitizing agent, trimethylpsoralin, binds to DNA as well as to melanin (22). The antimalarial compounds, quinacrine and chloroquine, bind to DNA (23) and pamaquine, a drug used to suppress the tissue form of the malaria parasites, is bound to a great extent to certain tissue proteins. Interestingly, a form of tissue binding interaction between pamaquin and quinacrine may occur. In the presence of quinacrine, the plasma concentrations of pamaquine are greatly increased. Doses of pamaquine which are normally tolerated when given alone are toxic in quinacrine treated patients (23).

It has been shown that chloroquine (24), phenothiazines (25), cocaine (26), and ephedrine (27) are concentrated in the pigmented structures of the eye. For each drug, the absence of comparable accumulation in nonpigmented (albino) tissue suggests that the melanin pigment (consisting mostly of indole polymers) is responsible for the binding of these drugs. This may explain why the mydriatic response to ephedrine was found to be inversely proportional to the degree of pigmentation of the iris (27).

Digoxin is relatively poorly bound to albumin, i.e. about 25 percent at therapeutic concentrations of 1 ng/ml (28), but shows strong affinity for a number of tissue macromolecules. In particular, cell membrane binding including interaction with the cardiac receptor, occurs largely with sodium/ potassium transport ATP'ase (29). Tissue binding of digoxin is strongest in the myocardium where steady-state tissue:serum ratios of 60 or greater have been found (29). In skeletal muscle, on the other hand, such ratios reach values of only about 15 (30).

Other tissue components which can bind drugs include calcified materials such as bone and teeth which show an appreciable affinity for the tetracyclines (31). Cationic drugs, such as quaternary ammonium compounds and amines, are bound to various degrees to acid mucopolysaccarides present in connective tissue. Kuntzman et al. (32) have shown that the nor-metabolites of two antihistaminic drugs, chlorcyclizine and cyclizine show strong affinity for tissue proteins. In particular, due to the strong affinity of norchlorcyclizine for tissue proteins, the latter was retained in the body long after the parent drug has disappeared.

Bickel and Steele (33) have examined the binding of a number of basic lipophilic drugs (chlorpromazine and imipramine) to cell fractions (microsomes, mitochondria). The interaction can be described by simple Scatchard-type binding with two classes of binding sites - one site of high affinity/low capacity and second site of low affinity/high capacity. In contrast to the basic lipophilic drugs, four acidic compounds (phenylbutazone, warfarin, salicylic acid and sulfadimethoxine) which bind strongly to serum albumin, show very weak or undetectable binding to liver fractions.

Bischoff, Dedrick and coworkers (34) have included parameters in their physiologic pharmacokinetic model for methotrexate which account for both linear nonspecific binding and strong saturable binding to dihydrofolate reductase.

Factors Which Alter Drug-Protein Binding

Protein Concentration

Many diseases and physiological alterations of the body cause changes in protein concentrations of the plasma and extravascular compartments. The interrelationship between percent binding, protein concentration, and drug concentration is nonlinear and complex. Figure 2 shows such behavior as calculated using mass-law principles. Drugs which are weakly bound ($K = 10^4$) show changes in binding which are somewhat proportional to the protein concentration, particularly over a physiological range of protein concentrations (10^{-5} to 10^{-3} M). The binding is only slightly different at the two concentrations of total drug in the system. The behavior of a drug with a strong association constant ($K = 10^7$) is the other extreme. Appreciable changes in protein concentration do not alter the degree of drug binding over an extensive range. However, at low concentrations of protein (less than 0.2×10^{-4} M), there is a substantial difference in binding which is dependent on the drug concentration. Drugs with an 'intermediate' association constant ($K = 10^5$) show appreciable dependence on both the drug and protein concentration in their degree of binding.

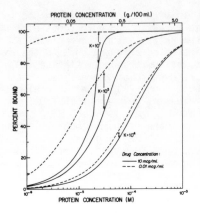

Fig 2. *Effect of protein concentration on the degree of binding of drugs with three different association constants and at two drug concentrations.*

The binding of dicloxacillin to albumin and to normal and uremic patient sera demonstrates this behavior (Figure 3) for a strongly bound antibiotic. Therefore, even though tissue concentrations of albumin and other binding macromolecules are often much less than that of plasma, the expected degree of drug binding can be appreciable depending on the association constant of the drug. Further studies of dicloxacillin binding in relation to molar ratio of free fatty acids to albumin are presented in Chapter 8.

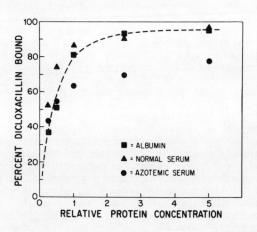

Fig. 3. *Relationship between percent binding of dicloxacillin and protein concentration (gm/dl albumin). Data are shown for human albumin, whole normal plasma, and pooled azotemic plasma.* (35)

Protein Concentration and Clinical Drug Effects and Disposition

There have been several published reports showing differences in clinical effects or pharmacokinetics which are related to serum protein concentrations. The Boston Collaborative Drug Surveillance Program has noted correlations between serum albumin levels and the frequency of side effects for three drugs: prednisone (36), phenytoin (37), and diazepam (38). In the case of diazepam, about 3 percent of patients with normal serum albumin concentrations (> 4.0 gm/dl) exhibited unwanted CNS depression. For patients with low serum albumin levels, the adverse reaction rate was as high as 9 percent. (The other drugs will be discussed in later sections.)

Azzollini et al. (39) have found that subjects with cirrhosis of the liver exhibit a slower elimination rate of chloramphenicol than normal subjects. They were able to show that the half-life of chloramphenicol was significantly correlated with the decrease in serum albumin and with an increase in serum bilirubin. This rather good correlation is probably the result of the fact that, at least for chloramphenicol, serum albumin levels are a good index of reduced drug-metabolizing activity on the part of hepatic microsomes. The same type of results have also been reported for amobarbital (40), aminopyrine (41), and phenylbutazone (42). Serum albumin concentration may thus serve as a marker for both liver dysfunction and perturbations in drug binding and distribution.

Effect of Diseases

Patients with impaired renal function have a high incidence of adverse drug reactions. Such drug reactions were originally thought to be mainly the result of decreased excretion of the drug by the kidneys leading to accumulation of the drug in the body. However, it is now well recognized that the binding capacity of many drugs is less in uremic patients than in normal subjects. Most of the drugs that show such abnormal binding are organic acids. Andreasen (43) has demonstrated decreased binding of six drugs (salicylic acid, acetylsalicylic acid, phenylbutazone, phenytoin, thiopental, and sulfadiazine) in patients suffering from acute renal failure caused by traffic accidents or complications of surgery. The plasma albumin concentration in these patients was below normal. However, even upon correction of the data for the albumin concentration, the binding capacity was still diminished. Reidenberg et al. (44) have found that binding of several basic drugs (quinidine, dapsone, and desmethylimipramine) is normal in uremic patients while binding of triamterene, also a basic drug, was decreased. A neutral compound, digitoxin, also has decreased binding in uremic plasma (45). Further studies comparing binding of sulfamethoxazole, dicloxacillin, phenytoin, salicylate, digitoxin, and penicillin G in sera from normal and uremic patients are described by Craig, Evenson, and Ramagopol in Chapter 8.

Reduced plasma protein binding of drugs is expected to result in a greater tissue distribution, a higher apparent volume of distribution, and a lower plasma concentration of the drug. Thus, uremic patients may respond to drug therapy at relatively lower total plasma concentrations than nonuremic patients. Letteri et al. (46), for example, have found that phenytoin concentrations are uniformly lower in uremic patients at the same dosage given to nonuremic patients. Uremic patients receiving 300 mg. phenytoin orally per day, exhibited an average plasma concentration of 4.44 µg/ml on the 14th day of therapy. Nonuremic patients, given the same dosage level, had plasma levels averaging 12.9 µg/ml. Odar-Cederlof et al. (47) have also reported that seizures disappeared in uremic patients at phenytoin plasma concentrations below the usual therapeutic range of 10-20 ug/ml. High (30%) unbound fractions of phenytoin were found in the uremic patients as compared with the lower unbound fractions (6-7%) in nonuremic patients. Decreased binding of phenytoin in uremia may be partly related to displacement of the drug from its binding sites by its metabolite, 5-phenyl-5-parahydroxylphenylhydantoin (HPPH). HPPH is not only strongly bound to albumin but also accumulates in the plasma to high levels in uremia (46).

Hyperlipoproteinemia, secondary to the presence of nephrotic syndrome, was the apparent cause of toxicity in six patients during therapy with the hypolipemic drug, clofibrate (48). A higher percentage of clofibrate (21-25%) was unbound in serum from these patients as compared with controls (3.1-8.2%). However, serum albumin concentrations were also reduced in these six patients which may partly cause reduced binding of clofibrate. Thus the dosage of clofibrate should be reduced in patients if the serum albumin concentration is low. (Clofibrate kinetics in rats where FFA concentrations were elevated by direct i.v. infusion have been discussed in Chapter 1.).

Plasma concentrations of free fatty acids (FFA) increase in patients with renal failure as a result of mobilization of adipose tissue (49). The affinity of FFA for albumin ($K = 10^7-10^8$) is greater than that of most drugs and, in sufficient quantity, FFA could be expected to compete for some of the drug binding sites on albumin. Rudman et al. (50) have found that in the concentration range normally seen in acute renal failure (2000-4000 μEq./L, 3.5-7.0 moles of FFA per mole of protein), FFA have a general inhibitory effect on the binding capacity of serum albumin with eight drugs (salicylate, phenytoin, phenylbutazone, sulfadiazine, thiopental, bishydroxycoumarin, bromosulfaphthalein, and octanoate). Fredholm et al. (51) used an *in situ* system where the subcutaneous adipose tissue of a dog is perfused with blood and sympathic nerve stimulation causes an increase in the free fatty acid concentration in blood. For phenytoin there was a linear relationship found between percent of drug free in blood and free fatty acid concentration. Gugler et al. (52) have also shown a good correlation between unbound concentrations of both warfarin and phenytoin and free fatty acid over a range of 750-800 μEq/L. A six-fold change in free concentration of warfarin and a two-fold change in free concentration of phenytoin were reported at a free fatty acid concentration of 2000 μEq/L. The degree of protein binding of phenytoin is shown to correlate well with the magnitude of the molar ratio of FFA:albumin in sera from eleven patients undergoing cardiopulmonary bypass procedures as presented in Chapter 8. Heparin, used during hemodialysis, activates lipoprotein lipase which results in a marked increase in the plasma levels of FFA and a reduction in drug binding capacity (53).

Altered binding of drugs occurs to a variable degree in cirrhosis. Affrime and Reidenberg examined four compounds (Table V) and found a small change in phenytoin binding while quinidine binding was markedly decreased. (Chapters 4 and 5 also describe changes in drug binding in liver disease.)

Cystic fibrosis causes hypoalbuminemia (15) and unusual serum protein is also formed (55). Jusko et al. (56) examined dicloxacillin binding in such patients as shown in Figure 4. While plasma binding was similar to normal in most cystic fibrosis subjects, the variability was appreciably greater in the cystic fibrosis patients and three out of thirteen patients had markedly decreased binding of the antibiotic.

Table V.   Drug Binding in Cirrhosis

	Percent Free	
	Normal	Cirrhotic
Fluorescein	13.8	25.6
Phenytoin	8.3	11.7
Quinidine	14.1	41.5
Triamterene	19.3	33.0

From Affrime & Reidenberg (54)

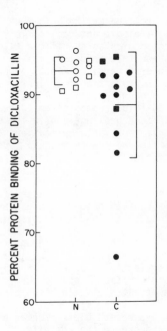

Fig. 4.   Plasma protein binding of dicloxacillin in 10 young healthy subjects (N) and in 13 adolescent patients with cystic fibrosis (C). The mean values and standard deviation are designated by horizontal lines.

The effect of gram-negative bacterial infection on FFA levels and binding of phenytoin is discussed in Chapter 8. Ascites appears to change the volume of distribution for propranolol without changes in the degree of protein binding as described in Chapter 5.

Structural Alterations of Proteins

Antibody formation or other drug-induced protein changes may result in an increased binding of drugs to serum. Aoyagi (57) has shown that, in patients allergic to para-aminosalicylic acid, binding is significantly higher than in nonallergic patients (Table VI). Ryan et al. (58) has noted a preferential binding of morphine to γ-globulin in addict sera in comparison with normal subjects. If the material injected by the addicts was antigenic, the greater affinity of morphine to addict sera may represent some degree of specific antibody binding.

Table VI. Protein Binding Of PAS In Allergic Patients

Percent Binding	Allergic:	No. of Patients NO	YES
20 - 29		7	1
30 - 39		21	2
40 - 49		7	1
50 - 59		3	6

From Aoyagi (57)

   Although there is much information regarding the function of antibodies as biologic antagonists to various macromolecules, the utilization of antibodies as specific antagonists to drugs is just beginning. It has been shown that injected anti-digoxin antibodies will protect rabbits from the adverse cardiac effects of an otherwise lethal dose of digoxin (59). Along with preventing intoxication, the anti-digoxin antibodies markedly alter the pharmacokinetics of digoxin. Antibody administration results in about a 100-fold greater serum concentration, decreased urinary excretion, and a 27-fold prolongation in the biologic half-life of digoxin. These studies have important implications in the field of drug toxicity. For example, Smith and coworkers have recently employed antibody fragments as an antidote to digoxin toxicity in one patient (60).

   One case report was recently published on the possibility of phenytoin-induced antibody formation (61). Although a large molecular weight material is usually needed to cause antibody production, prolonged drug usage may lead to antibody induction in a small number of patients.

   Another type of drug-induced change in protein binding is the acetylation of albumin. For example, the acetyl group of aspirin can become covalently attached to the lysine of albumin (62), thus causing a conformational change that affects the binding of other drugs. The acetylated albumin has a higher affinity for phenylbutazone and a lower affinity for flufenamic acid (63). Many drugs (3) have also been shown to cause reversible conformational changes in albumin which may either increase or decrease the affinity of other drugs to albumin.

   The occurrence of an unusual serum protein in cystic fibrosis patients (55) and the modification of the serum albumin molecule in patients with rheumatoid arthritis (64) are two other disease associated modifications of protein structure. No pharmacokinetic implications of these effects are known.

Effect Of Binding On Disposition Of Specific Drugs

Physiological Pharmacokinetics

   Physiological pharmacokinetic models have been successfully used to describe the distribution and elimination of thiopental (65), methotrexate (34), arabinosyl cytosine (66), and lidocaine (67). All parameters used in such models have a specific physiologic or physicochemical basis. They thereby provide a more realistic basis for considering the handling of drugs

110

by the body than the methods used in conventional compartmental pharmacokinetics. This section utilizes a physiologic pharmacokinetic model to simulate the expected pharmacokinetic effects of varying albumin binding.

The type of physiologic pharmacokinetic model which was used includes body regions such as shown in Figure 5. In particular, each tissue region is separated into three water compartments: The capillary plasma volume, the interstitial water, and the intracellular water. Each major organ or tissue region receives a designated plasma flow. The numerical parameters and the mathematics of this type of system have been described previously (68) and are essentially adapted from the work of Bischoff and Dedrick (34). For simplicity, red cell uptake of the drug was ignored and linear binding of the drug to albumin was assumed to occur in both the plasma and interstitial space. The plasma and tissue albumin concentrations are realistic with the plasma and liver interstitial protein concentration set at 5.0×10^{-4}M, the central nervous system value set at zero, and all other interstitial fluids given values one-half of the plasma protein concentration. An adipose:plasma water partition coefficient of 100 was used. The only route of elimination of this hypothetical drug was considered to be metabolism in the liver with an hepatic rate constant of 0.8 min^{-1}. Association constants (K) for binding to albumin of 10^4, 10^5 and 10^7 were examined.

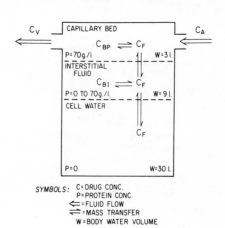

Fig. 5. *Tissue or organ section of a physiological pharmacokinetic model showing equilibration of the unbound drug (C_F) between water compartments and binding with proteins (C_B).*

The MIMED computer program (69) for numerical integration was used to simulate two distinct cases. In one case it was assumed that the metabolic rate constant was acting on the total drug concentration in the liver, (Case I) and in the other case the metabolic rate constant was acting only on the free concentration of the drug in the liver (Case II).

The effects of the two metabolic conditions on the time course of plasma drug concentrations after a single 10 mg. dose are shown in Figures 6 and 7. In addition, numerical values for several model-independent pharmacokinetic parameters derived from the simulation are listed on the figures. In both

111

cases the steady-state volume of distribution (V_D^{ss}) changes in inverse relation to the association constant. As binding increases more of the drug is located in the plasma relative to the rest of the body, resulting in a decrease in the steady-state volume of distribution. The similarities of the two cases cease at this point. In Case I, increased binding accelerates the rate of elimination ($t_{1/2\beta}$ decreases) because more drug becomes available to the site of metabolism. However, Case II is more complex. At the same time as more total drug is becoming available to the liver, the fraction of this quantity which is free and therefore available for metabolism is decreasing. Thus one notes an initial decrease in $t_{1/2\beta}$ and then an increase in $t_{1/2\beta}$ as the extent of binding increases further. In Case I there is little change in the metabolic clearance (CL_m) as the extent of binding changes while in Case II, CL_m decreases as the extent of binding increases. Since the steady-state drug concentration and CL_m are inversely related, as the extent of binding increases the steady-state plasma levels are expected to increase markedly in Case II, while Case I will show only a small increase.

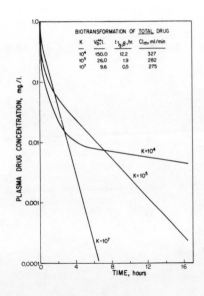

Fig. 6. *Effect of plasma protein binding (3 association constants) on the hypothetical pharmacokinetics of a drug described by a physiological model. It is assumed that the metabolic rate constant is acting on the total drug concentration in the liver (Case I). Some model independent pharmacokinetic parameters are listed on the figure for each binding constant.*

It appears from these simulations that the distributional characteristics of a drug are quite similar in both cases being related to protein binding (among other factors). However the mechanism of hepatic availability of a drug has a profound effect on the disposition behavior of a drug. The *type* of phenomena as Case I has been proposed to account for differences in the pharmacokinetics of propranolol among subjects (70). On the other hand, the elimination rate of the anticoagulants, warfarin and dicoumarol, as well as phenytoin appears to be determined by the free drug concentration in plasma and liver (71) and data are observed which resemble Case II.

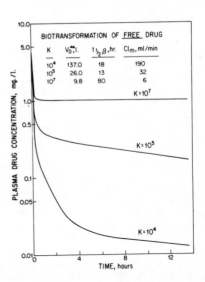

Fig. 7. *Effect of plasma protein binding (3 association constants) on the hypothetical pharmacokinetics of a drug described by a physiological model. It is assumed that the metabolic rate constant is acting on only the free drug concentration in the liver (Case II).*

The present simulation was limited to examining the effects of the availability of *free* versus *total* drug in the liver. An analogous phenomenon occurs in the kidney. The glomerular filtration rate of a drug is determined by the *free* drug concentration in plasma whereas the process of tubular secretion acts upon *total* drug presented to the kidney. Since most drugs have more than one route and mechanism of elimination, the relationship between protein binding and pharmacokinetic behavior can be considerably more complex. The renal mechanism of excretion (glomerular filtration, tubular secretion, tubular reabsorption, or a combination of these) is usually known for many drugs. With the exception of a few drugs, it is not known whether only *free* drug or *total* drug is available to the drug metabolizing enzymes. Other factors such as lipid partitioning and additional tissue binding will further complicate the pharmacokinetic picture.

Phenytoin Binding

Phenytoin (DPH) has been one of the most comprehensively studied drugs with respect to the clinical role of and factors affecting its binding to plasma proteins. At therapeutic serum concentrations, the drug is bound largely to albumin and partly to α-globulins to the degree of 85 to 95 percent in healthy human subjects (72). Distribution of the drug into tissues is partly controlled by protein binding in that there is a close correlation between unbound DPH in plasma and concentrations in CSF fluid (73), in erythrocytes (74), and in saliva (75) over an appreciable range of concentrations. In fact, Viukari and Tammisto found that, in relation to control of seizures, there is less scatter in the range of DPH concentrations found in CSF than in the serum (76). This suggests that more variability occurs in serum binding of DPH than in CSF distribution.

As pointed out previously, the protein binding of DPH in plasma is decreased in uremia (77) and in the presence of FFA (52). However,

113

hyperbilirubinemia (78), fetal serum (79), nephrosis (80), and
hypoalbuminemia (81) also diminish the binding of the anticonvulsant. The
decreased binding of DPH produces lower plasma concentrations and a larger
apparent volume of distribution of the drug in uremic patients (46). The
Boston Collaborative Drug Surveillance Program has shown that hypoalbuminemia
is associated with an increased incidence of adverse reactions to DPH in
treated patients (37). Drugs often administered to epileptic or cardiac
patients such as salicylate, sulfisoxazole, phenylbutazone, and acetazolamide
displace DPH from plasma proteins (81) and are a potential source of drug
interactions.

Therapeutic plasma concentrations of DPH usually range from 10 to 20 mg/L
but differences in protein binding can cause patients to require higher or
lower levels of the drug for an adequate and nontoxic effect. Booker and
Darcey found that the unbound concentration of DPH in plasma provides a much
better discrimination between toxic and nontoxic patients than total plasma
concentrations of the drug. Their findings are shown in Figure 8 (82).

The data of Booker and Darcey and the host of drug and disease factors
which are capable of altering the plasma protein binding of DPH suggests that
the measurement of unbound, rather than total, plasma concentrations of DPH
may be a better method of monitoring the therapeutic use of the anticonvulsant. Two approaches to overcoming the time-consuming maneuvers of
directly measuring DPH protein binding by either ultrafiltration or
equilibrium dialysis is to take advantage of either saliva or erythrocyte
concentrations of the drug. Both saliva (83) and erythrocyte (84)
concentrations of DPH are proportional to the unbound concentration of
anticonvulsant in plasma.

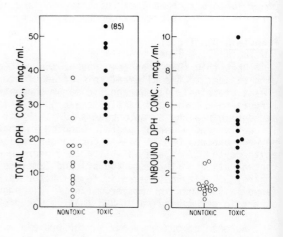

Fig. 8.   Effect of protein
          binding of phenytoin
          on the relationship
          between serum
          concentrations and
          toxicity in treated
          patients. Data are
          from Reference 82.

114

Corticosteroid Binding

The protein binding of corticosteroids is of physiologic importance because it appears that the circulating free concentration of the steroids is responsible for biochemical and pharmacologic effects on the body as well as control of the adrenal cortical system (85). Many steroids are bound not only to albumin but also to specific α- and β-globulins present in plasma. Corticosteroid binding globulin (CBG, transcortin) shows a high affinity for steroids such as cortisol, corticosterone and prednisolone. Recently, a β-globulin named gonadal binding globulin (GBG), has been identified as strongly binding testosterone and estradiol (86). Although these α and β globulins have high affinity for specific steroids, their relatively low concentrations in plasma ($\sim 10^{-7}$M), cause saturation in binding as the steroid concentration is increased above physiological levels. This is demonstrated by the data for prednisolone in Figure 9. Cortisol behaves similarly.

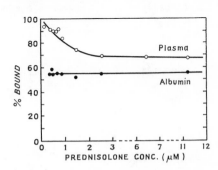

Fig. 9. Binding of prednisolone to pooled human plasma and to 3.5% human albumin solution. Data are from Lewis et al. (36).

Although albumin has a lower affinity constant, it has a greater capacity to bind steroids because of its relatively larger plasma concentration ($\sim 10^{-4}$M). These factors cause the distribution of steroids to differ at physiologic and pharmacologic doses. Cortisol, for example, at physiologic doses of 270 μg - 500 μg has a volume of distribution ranging from 9.5 - 17 liters in man (87). At pharmacologic doses of 50-500 mg, the volume of distribution of cortisol is about 70-80 liters in man (88). Similar effects can be noted for prednisolone from the data of Meickle et al. (89) as shown in Table VII. These binding and distribution differences lead to changes in the half-life and metabolic clearance of both cortisol and prednisolone.

Table VII. Effect Of Dose On Prednisolone Disposition

Dose, mg	V_D L./m^2	$t_{1/2}$, min.	CL L./day/m^2
12	19.5	240	82
48	34.0	300	100

From Meickle et al. (89)

A pharmacokinetic rationalization of the effects of saturation in CBG binding of prednisolone in man has been developed by Lewis et al. (36). A model, similar to the one shown in Figure 5, was constructed to examine the role of plasma and interstitial CBG and albumin on prednisolone distribution under steady-state conditions. It was found that prednisolone binding and distribution would be affected by both the dose of the steroid and the concentration of the proteins. These simulations were used to explain, in part, the findings of the Boston Collaborative Drug Surveillance Program (36) that the incidence of adverse reactions from prednisone (a pro-drug of prednisolone) were markedly higher in patients with low serum albumin concentrations (Table VIII).

Table VIII. Frequency Of Side Effects From Prednisone In Relation To Dose And Serum Albumin Concentration

Mean Daily Dose, mg	Serum Albumin gm/dl	No. of Patients	Percent With Side Effects
1-25	≤ 2.5	11	9
	≥ 2.6	84	12
25-50	≤ 2.5	11	36
	≥ 2.6	71	14
50+	≤ 2.5	13	62
	≥ 2.6	50	20

From Lewis et al. (36)

Digoxin Binding

The plasma protein binding of digoxin is of little importance in affecting the pharmacokinetics of this cardiac glycoside. Normal adults (90) bind only 18 to 33 percent of the drug in plasma (mean = 25.2%). However, the interaction of digoxin with tissue binding sites appears to be a major factor which determines the relatively large volume of distribution (V_β^{ss}) of the drug as well as its variability in disposition in patients with renal impairment. In particular, digoxin binds to sodium/potassium transport ATP'ase enzymes in the cell membrane as its major tissue interaction site (91) with additional binding occurring with intracellular soluble proteins (92) and with the contractile proteins, actin and myosin (93). Tissue binding is strongest in the myocardium where steady-state tissue:serum concentration ratios of 60 or greater are found in adults with normal renal function (29).

Azotemic patients exhibit unusual distribution characteristics for digoxin. The myocardium:serum concentration ratio for digoxin decreases as renal function (creatinine clearance) falls, indicative of diminished tissue uptake of the drug (Figure 10). This distributional change corresponds with the differences in V_β^{ss} observed between normal and renal failure patients. Uremic patients have V_β^{ss} values which average about 60 percent of normal (29). The effect of uremia on digoxin distribution is consistent with findings of Kramer et al. (94) that Na/K ATP'ase enzyme activity is inhibited in uremic rats.

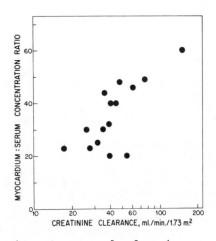

Fig. 10. *Relationship of the*
myocardial:serum
concentration ratio of
digoxin at autopsy to
the estimated premorbid
creatinine clearance of
15 patients. Data are
from Jusko and Weintraub
(29).

Infants also exhibit unusual dosage requirements, serum levels and pharmacokinetics of digoxin which may be partly related to tissue distribution and binding. The maintenance dose of digoxin is about 400-600 $\mu g/m^2$ in infants at about 3 months of age while adults require 140-300 $\mu g/m^2$. The usual therapeutic range of digoxin serum levels is about 0.7 to 1.5 ng/ml in adults, while infants are usually maintained on serum levels of 2 to 4 ng/ml. The V_D^{ss} values of digoxin in adults averages about 7.1 L/kg (95) while infants exhibit values of 16.2 L./kg (96). We examined myocardium:serum distribution ratios in autopsy specimens from infants and a comparison of the results with adult data are shown in Figure 11 (97). Myocardial uptake of digoxin was nearly twice as great in infants as in adults at any given serum concentration. These findings are consistent with a greater apparent value of distribution of digoxin in infants and may partly explain the unusually large therapeutic doses needed in infants. There appear to be two types of equilibria between serum and myocardial concentrations of digoxin. Total tissue uptake, which reflects overall binding and generalized distribution of digoxin, and the serum-receptor equilibrium which allows serum levels to serve as a proportionality factor in determining the therapeutic and toxic effects of the cardiac glycoside (29).

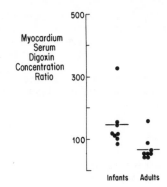

Fig. 11. *Myocardium:serum concentration*
ratio of digoxin in infants
and adults. Data are from
Gorodischer et al. (97).

117

Summary

Plasma and tissue proteins are the major interface for pharmacokinetic interaction of drugs in the body. The binding of drugs to proteins and the resulting pharmacokinetics of the compound can be modified in disease states which alter either the concentration of proteins or the biophysical/biochemical nature of the macromolecules, as well as in pathological conditions which cause accumulation of endogenous materials capable of displacing drugs from binding sites on the protein.

Macromolecules which interact with drugs include: albumin, various globulins, ligandin, cell membranes, mucopolysaccharides, DNA, bone, collagen, melanin, and various specific drug receptors. Albumin is the major soluble protein accounting for nonspecific drug binding in the body. About 140 grams of albumin are found in plasma and about 180 grams are distributed throughout the interstitial fluids at various concentrations in man. There is a complex, nonlinear relationship between drug binding and protein concentration which is also dependent on the drug-protein association constant and drug concentration.

Pathological conditions which reduce albumin levels in the body include: acute factors such as burns, freezing, bone fractures, myocardial infarction, surgery, and febrile infections, and chronic conditions such as neoplastic disease, malnutrition, liver impairment, renal disease (especially nephrosis), some gastrointestinal disorders, bronchitis, and cystic fibrosis. Elevated serum albumin concentrations are rare, occurring most often in patients with psychological disorders.

Several factors may cause structural changes in proteins. These include: acetylation of albumin by aspirin, occurrence of an unique form of albumin in rheumatoid arthritis, and apparent antibody formation to some drugs.

Accumulation of endogenous compounds capable of displacing drugs from protein binding sites occurs in renal disease, in hyperbilirubinemia, and in conditions causing increased FFA levels. The combined effect of hypoproteinemia and increased FFA reduces drug binding in patients with renal disease.

A physiologic pharmacokinetic model was used to simulate the effect of protein binding on the disposition kinetics of drugs. While binding directly affects the V_D^S of drugs, the rate of drug elimination is dependent on whether free or total drug can be removed by excretory/metabolic enzymes.

Three drugs whose clinical effects and disposition kinetics are determined by plasma or tissue binding are phenytoin, prednisolone, and digoxin.

Acknowledgments

Supported in part by Grant No. 20852 from the National Institutes of General Medical Sciences of the NIH. The secretarial assistance of Ms. Sheryln Sion is greatly appreciated.

References

1. M. A. Rothschild, A. Bauman, R. S. Yalow and S. A. Berson. Tissue distribution of I^{131} labeled human serum albumin following intravenous administration. J. Clin. Invest. 34:1354-1358 (1955).
2. M. A. Rothschild, M. Oratz and S. S. Schreiber. Albumin metabolism. Gastroenterology 64:324-337 (1973).
3. W. J. Jusko and M. Gretch. Plasma and tissue protein binding of drugs in pharmacokinetics. Drug Met. Rev. 5:in press (1976).
4. A. E. Casey, F. E. Gilbert, H. Copeland, E. L. Downey and J. G. Casey. Albumin, alpha-1,-2, beta and gamma globulin in cancer and other diseases. Southern Med. J. 66:179-185 (1973).
5. L. O. Plantin, S. Ahlinder, R. Norberg and G. Birke. The distribution of proteins between intra and extravascular spaces in health and disease. Acta Med. Scand. 189:309-314 (1971).
6. D. Casten, M. Bodenhumer and J. Burcham. A study of plasma protein variation in surgical procedure. Ann. Surg. 117:52-73 (1943).
7. G. Birke, S. O. Liljedahl, L. O. Plantin and J. Wetterfors. Albumin catabolism in burns and following surgical procedures. Acta Chir. Scandinav. 118:353-366 (1959-1960).
8. W. Gleichmann, G. W. Backmann, H. J. Dengler and J. Dudeck. Effect of hormonal contraceptives and pregnancy on serum protein pattern. Europ. J. Clin. Pharmacol. 5:218-225 (1973).
9. G. B. Midler, E. L. Alling and J. J. Morton. Effect of neoplastic and allied diseases on concentration of plasma proteins. Cancer 3:56-65 (1950).
10. J. L. Steinfeld. I^{131}-Albumin degradation in patients with neoplastic diseases. Cancer 13:974-984 (1960).
11. S. Skrede, J. P. Blomhoff, K. Elgjo and E. Gjone. Serum proteins in diseases of the liver. Scand. J. Clin. Lab. Invest. 35:399-406 (1975).
12. H. Jensen, N. Rossing, S. B. Andersen and S. Jarnum. Albumin metabolism in the nephrotic syndrome in adults. Clin. Sci. 33:445-457 (1967).
13. M. A. Rothschild, M. Oratz and S. S. Schreiber. Albumin synthesis. NEJM 286:816-821 (1972).
14. L. Bonomo and A. D'Addabbo. I^{131} Albumin turnover and loss of proteins into the sputum in chronic bronchitis. Clin. Chim. Acta. 10:214-222 (1964).
15. W. Strober, G. Peter and R. H. Schwartz. Albumin metabolism in cystic fibrosis. Pediatrics 43:416-426 (1969).
16. E. A. Casey, F. E. Gilbert, J. F. Gravlce and E. L. Downey. Low urea-nitrogen and elevated serum albumin in anxiety, neuroses, and psychoses. Alabama J. Med. Sci. 8:168-177 (1971).
17. B. Ecanow, B. H. Gold and P. Tunkunas. Serum albumin and urea during states of anxiety and depression. J.A.M.A. 226:356 (1973).
18. G. Litwack, B. Ketterer and I. M. Arias. Ligandin: A hepatic protein which binds steroids, bilirubin, carcinogens, and a number of exogenous organic anious. Nature 234:466-467 (1971).
19. R. Corrocher, G. DeSandre, M. L. Pacor and A. V. Hoffbrand. Hepatic protein binding of folate. Clin. Sci. Mol. Med. 46:551-554 (1974).
20. D. R. Davis and R. A. Yeary. Bilirubin binding to hepatic Y and Z protein (Ligandin): Tissue bilirubin concentration in phenobarbital treated gunn rat. Proc. Soc. Exp. Biol. Med. 148:9-13 (1975).

21. L. M. Allen and P. J. Creaven. Binding of a new antitumor agent, thalicarpine to DNA. J. Pharm. Sci. 63:474-475 (1974).
22. M. S. Blois and L. Taskovich. The reversible binding of some aromatic and cyclic compounds to biopolymers in vitro. J. Invest. Dermatology 53:344-350 (1969).
23. N. B. Kurnick and I. E. Radcliffe. Reaction between DNA and quinacrine and other antimalarials. J. Lab. Clin. Med. 60:669-688 (1962).
24. H. Bernstein, N. Zvaifler, M. Rubin and A. M. Mansour. The ocular deposition of chloroquine. Invest. Ophthalmol. 2:384-392 (1963).
25. A. Potts. The concentration of phenothiazines in the eye of experimental animals. Invest. Ophthalmol. 1:522-530 (1962).
26. P. N. Patil. Cocaine-binding by the pigmented and the non-pigmented iris and its relevance to the mydriatic effect. Invest. Ophthalmol. 11:739-746 (1972).
27. P. N. Patil, K. Shimada, D. R. Feller and L. Malspeis. Accumulation of $(-)-^{14}C$-ephedrine by the pigmented and the non-pigmented iris. J. Pharmacol. Exp. Therap. 188:342-352 (1974).
28. D. S. Lukas and A. G. DeMartino. Binding of digitoxin and some related cardenolides to human plasma proteins. J. Clin. Invest. 48:1041-1053 (1969).
29. W. J. Jusko and M. Weintraub. Myocardial distribution of digoxin and renal function. Clin. Pharmacol. Ther. 16:449-454 (1974).
30. J. E. Doherty, W. H. Perkins and W. J. Flanigan. The distribution and concentration of tritiated digoxin in human tissues. Ann. Int. Med. 66:116-124 (1967).
31. R. G. Kelly and L. A. Kanegis. Tissue distribution of tetracycline and chlortetracycline in the dog. Toxicol. Appl. Pharmacol. 11:114-120 (1967).
32. R. Kuntzman, M. Jacobson, I. Tsai, J. J. Burns, J. Burchall and A. Kock. Certain aspects of drug binding to non-plasma proteins as illustrated by studies with cyclizine, chlorcyclizine and polymyxin B. Ann. NY Acad. Sci. 226: (1973).
33. M. H. Bickel and J. W. Steele. Binding of basic and acidic drugs to rat tissue subcellular fractions. Chem-Biol. Interactions 8:151-162 (1974).
34. K. B. Bischoff, R. L. Dedrick, D. S. Zahahko and J. A. Longstreth. Methotrexate pharmacokinetics. J. Pharm. Sci. 60:1128 (1971).
35. W. J. Jusko, L. M. Gerbracht and M. L. Rocci. Effect of protein binding on β-lactamase inactivation of penicillins, Presented at the Academy of Pharmaceutical Sciences meeting, New Orleans, Nov. (1975).
36. G. P. Lewis, C. W. Burke, L. Graves and W. J. Jusko. Prednisone side effects and serum protein levels. Lancet 778-781 (1971) (Oct. 9).
37. Boston Collaborative Drug Surveillance Program, Boston, MA, Boston University Medical Center. Diphenylhydantoin side effects and serum albumin levels, Clin. Pharmacol. Ther. 14:529-532 (1973).
38. D. J. Greenblatt and J. Koch-Weser. Clinical toxicity of chlordiazepoxide and diazepam in relation to serum albumin concentration: A report from the Boston Collaborative Drug Surveillance Program. Europ. J. Clin. Pharmacol. 7:259-262 (1974).
39. F. Azzollini, A. Gazzaniga, E. Lodola and R. Natangelo. Elimination of chloramphenicol and thiamphenicol in subjects with cirrhosis of the liver. Int. J. Clin. Pharmacol. 6:130-134 (1972).
40. G. E. Mawer, N. E. Miller and L. A. Turnberg. Metabolism of amylobarbitone in patients with chronic liver disease. Brit. J. Pharmacol. 44:549-560 (1972).

41. G. W. Hepner and E. S. Vesell. Quantitative assessment of hepatic function by breath analysis after oral administration of [^{14}C] aminopyrine. Ann. Intern. Med. 83:632-638 (1975).
42. A. J. Levi, S. Sherlock and D. Walker. Phenylbutazone and isoniazid metabolism in patients with liver disease in relation to previous drug therapy, Lancet I:1275-1279 (1968).
43. F. Andreasen. Protein binding of drugs in plasma from patients with acute renal failure. Acta. Pharmacol. et. Toxicol. 32:417-429 (1973).
44. M. M. Reidenberg and M. Affrime. Influence of disease on binding of drugs to plasma proteins. Ann. NY Acad. Sci. 226: (1973).
45. D. W. Shoeman and D. L. Azarnoff. The alteration of plasma proteins in uremia as reflected in their ability to bind digitoxin and diphenylhydantoin. Pharmac. 7:169-177 (1972).
46. J. M. Letteri, H. Mellk, S. Louis, H. Kutt, P. Durante and A. Glazko. Diphenylhydantoin metabolism in uremia. N. Eng. J. Med. 285:648 (1971).
47. I. Odar-Cederlöf, Per Lunde and Folke Sjöqvist. Abnormal Pharmacokinetics of phenytoin in a patient with uremia. Lancet 831 (1970).
48. J. G. Bridgeman, S. M. Rosen and J. M. Thorp. Complication during clofibrate treatment of nephrotic-syndrome hyperlipoproteinemia. Lancet 506 (1972).
49. M. S. Losowsky and D. H. Kenward. Lipid metabolism in acute and chronic renal failure. J. Lab. Clin. Med. 71:736 (1968).
50. D. Rudman, T. J. Bixler and A. E. Del Rio. Effects of FFA on binding of drugs by bovine serum albumin, by human serum albumin, and by rabbit serum. J. Pharmac. Exp. Therap. 176:261 (1971).
51. B. B. Fredholm, A. Rane and B. Persson. Diphenylhydantoin binding to proteins in plasma and its dependence on free fatty acids and bilirubin concentration in dog and newborn infants. Pediatric Res. 9:26-30 (1975).
52. R. Gugler, D. W. Shoeman and D.L. Azarnoff. Effect of in vivo elevation of free fatty acids on protein binding of drugs. Pharmacol. 12:160-165 (1974).
53. S. H. Dromgoole. The effects of hemodialysis on the binding capacity of albumin. Clin. Chim. Acta. 46:469-472 (1973).
54. M. Affrime and M. Reidenberg. The protein binding of some drugs in plasma from patients with alcoholic liver disease. Europ. J. Clin. Pharmacol. 8:267-269 (1975).
55. G. B. Wilson, T. L. Jahn and J. R. Fonseca. Demonstration of serum protein differences in cystic fibrosis by isoelectric focusing in thin-layer polyacrylamide gels. Clin. Chim. Acta. 49:79-91 (1973).
56. W. J. Jusko, L. L. Mosovich, L. M. Gerbracht, M. E. Mattar and S. J. Yaffe. Enhanced renal excretion of dicloxacillin in patients with cystic fibrosis. Pediatrics 56:1038-1044 (1975).
57. T. Aoyagi. Protein binding of rifampicin to different individual sera. Scand. J. Resp. Dis. Suppl. 84:44-49 (1973).
58. J. J. Ryan, C. W. Parker and R. C. Williams. γ-globulin binding of morphine in heroin addicts. J. Lab. Clin. Med. 80:155-164 (1972).
59. D. H. Schmidt and V. P. Butler. Immunological protection against digoxin toxicity. J. Clin. Invest. 50:866-871 (1971).
60. T. W. Smith, E. Haber, L. Yeatman and V. P. Butler. Reversal of advanced digoxin intoxication with FAB fragments of digoxin-specific antibodies. N. Engl. J. Med. 294:797-800 (1976).
61. H. B. Kleckner. Severe hypersensitivity to diphenylhydantoin with circulating antibodies to drugs. Ann. Intern. Med. 83: 522 (1975).

62. D. Hawkins, R. N. Pinckard and R. S. Farr. Acetylation of human serum albumin by acetylsalicylic acid. Science 160:780-781 (1968).
63. R. S. Farr, R. T. Reid and P. Minden. Spontaneous and induced alterations in the anion-binding properties of human albumin. J. Clin. Invest. 45:1006 (1966).
64. R. T. Reid and R. S. Farr. Further evidence for albumin alterations in some patients with rheumatic disease. Arthritis Rheum. 7:747-748 (1964).
65. K. B. Bischoff and R. L. Dedrick. Thiopental pharmacokinetics. J. Pharm. Sci. 57:1346-1351 (1968).
66. R. L. Dedrick, D. D. Forrester and D. H. W. Ho. In vitro-in vivo correlation of drug metabolism-deamination of 1-β-Arabino-furanosylcytosine. Biochem. Pharmacol. 21:1-16 (1972).
67. N. Benowitz, R. P. Forsyth, K. L. Melmon and M. Rowland. Lidocaine disposition kinetics in monkey and man. I. Prediction by a perfusion model. Clin. Pharmacol. Ther. 16:87-98 (1974).
68. W. J. Jusko. Factors affecting the pharmacokinetics of some psychoactive drugs, In E. M. Sellers (ed.), Clinical Pharmacology of Psychoactive Drugs, Alcoholism and Drug Addiction Research Foundation, Toronto, 1975, pp. 55-71.
69. MIMED, State University of New York at Buffalo Office of Computer Services adaptation of MIMIC. A Digital Simulation Language, Control Data Corporation, St. Paul, Minn., 1968.
70. G. H. Evans and D. G. Shand. Disposition of propranolol VI, Independent variation in steady-state circulating drug concentration and half-life as a result of plasma drug binding in man. Clin. Pharmacol. Ther. 14:494 (1973).
71. G. Levy. Relationship between plasma protein binding, distribution, and anticoagulant action of dicumarol. Ann. NY Acad. Sci. 226:195-199 (1973).
72. A. J. Glazko and T. Chang. Diphenylhydantoin: Absorption, distribution, and excretion, In D. M. Woodbury, J. K. Penry and R. P. Schmidt, (eds.), Antiepileptic Drugs, Raven Press, New York, (1972), 127-136.
73. L. Lund, A. Berlin and P. K. M. Lunde. Plasma protein binding of diphenylhydantoin in patients with epilepsy. Agreement between the unbound fraction in plasma and the concentration in the cerebrospinal fluid. Clin. Pharmacol. Ther. 13:196-200 (1972).
74. P. Borondy, W. A. Dill, T. Change, R. A. Buchanan and A. J. Glazko. Effect of protein binding on the distribution of 5,5-diphenylhydantoin between plasma and red cells. Ann. NY Acad. Sci. 226:82-87 (1973).
75. O. Svensmark, P. J. Schiller and F. Buchtal. 5,5-diphenylhydantoin (Dilantin) blood levels after oral or intravenous dosage in man. Acta. Pharmacol. et. Toxicol. 16:331-346 (1960).
76. N. M. A. Viukari and P. Tammisto. Diphenylhydantoin as an anti-convulsant: Protein binding and fluctuation of the serum and CSF levels in 40 mentally subnormal epileptics. J. Ment. Defec. Res. 13:235-244 (1969).
77. M. M. Reidenberg, I. Odar-Cederlof, C. von Bahr, O. Borga and F. Sjoqvist. Protein binding of diphenylhydantoin and desmethylimipramine in plasma from patients with poor renal function. N. Engl. J. Med. 285:264-267 (1971).
78. A. Rane, P. K. M. Lunde, B. Jalling, S. J. Yaffe and F. Sjoqvist. Plasma protein binding of diphenylhydantoin in normal and hyper-bilirubinemic infants. J. Ped. 78:877-882 (1971).

79. A. W. Pruitt and P. G. Dayton. A comparison of the binding of drugs to adult and cord plasma. Europ. J. Clin. Pharmacol. 4:59-62 (1971).
80. R. Gugler, D. W. Shoeman, D. H. Huffman, J. B. Cohlmia and D. L. Azarnoff. Pharmacokinetics of drugs in patients with the nephrotic syndrome. J. Clin. Invest. 55:1182-1189 (1975).
81. P. K. M. Lunde, A. Rene, S. J. Yaffe, L. Lund and F. Sjoqvist. Plasma protein binding of diphenylhydantoin in man. Interaction with other drugs and the effect of temperature and plasma dilution. Clin. Pharmacol. Ther. 11:846-855 (1970).
82. H. E. Booker and B. Darcey. Serum concentrations of free diphenylhydantoin and their relationship to clinical intoxication. Epilepsia 14:177-184 (1973).
83. F. Bochner, W. D. Hooper, J. M. Sutherland, M. J. Eadie and J. H. Tyrer. Diphenylhydantoin concentrations in saliva. Arch. Neurol. 31:57-59 (1974).
84. D. Kurata and G. R. Wilkinson. Erythrocyte uptake and plasma binding of diphenylhydantoin. Clin. Pharmacol. Ther. 16:355-362 (1974).
85. F. E. Yates, R. D. Brennan and J. Urquhart. Adrenal glucocorticoid control system. Fed. Proc. 28:71-83 (1969).
86. L. M. Sherwood and E. E. Parris. Interaction of adrenal and gonadal steroids with proteins in human plasma. N. Engl. J. Med. 281:658-665 (1969).
87. R. E. Peterson and J. B. Wyngaarden. The miscible pool and turnover rate of hydrocortisone in man. J. Clin. Invest. 35:552-561 (1956).
88. R. E. Peterson, J. B. Wyngaarden, S. L. Guerra, B. B. Brodie and J. J. Bunim. The physiological disposition and metabolic fate of hydrocortisone in man. J. Clin. Invest. 34:1779-1794 (1955).
89. A. W. Meikle, J. A. Weed and F. H. Tyler. Kinetics of interconversion of prednisolone and prednisone studied with new radioimmunoassays, J. Clin. Endocrin. Met. 41:717-721 (1975).
90. J. R. Koup, W. J. Jusko, C. M. Elwood and R. K. Kohli. Digoxin pharmacokinetics: Role of renal failure in dosage regimen design. Clin. Pharmacol. Ther. 18:9-21 (1975).
91. R. Thomas. Enzymes as drug receptors: Transport ATPase. Austral. J. Pharm. Sci. NS1:9-15 (1972).
92. T. Godfraind and M. Lesne. The uptake of cardiac glycosides in relation to their actions in isolated cardiac muscle. Brit. J. Pharmacol. 46:488-497 (1972).
93. E. Genazzani and R. Santamaria. Interaction of cardiac glycosides with serum albumin and contractile proteins. Pharmacol. Res. Comm. 1: 249-257 (1969).
94. H. J. Kramer, A. Backer and F. Kruck. Inhibition of intestinal (Na+-K+)-ATPase in experimental uremia. Clin. Chim. Acta. 50:13-18 (1974).
95. J. R. Koup, D. J. Greenblatt, W. J. Jusko, T. W. Smith and J. Koch-Weser. Pharmacokinetics of digoxin in normal subjects after intravenous bolus and infusion doses. J. Pharmacok. Biopharm. 3:181-192 (1975).
96. P. L. Morselli, B. M. Assael, R. Gomeni, M. Mandelli, A. Marini, E. Reali, U. Visconti and F. Sereni. Digoxin pharmacokinetics during human development. In P. L. Morselli, S. Garanttini and F. Sereni (eds.), Basic and Therapeutic Aspects of Perinatal Pharmacology, Raven Press, New York, 1975, pp. 377-392.
97. R. Gorodischer, W. J. Jusko and S. J. Yaffe. Tissue and erythrocyte distribution of digoxin in infants. Clin. Pharmacol. Ther. 19:256-262 (1976).

Chapter 8

THE EFFECT OF UREMIA, CARDIOPULMONARY BYPASS AND

BACTERIAL INFECTION ON SERUM PROTEIN BINDING

William A. Craig, Merle A. Evenson and V. Ramgopal

Serum protein binding appears to be one of the important determinants of drug distribution in the body. Highly bound drugs tend to remain in the vascular compartment, while slightly bound drugs may diffuse more readily into the interstitial fluid. The effect of disease states on protein binding has only recently been appreciated. For example, as discussed in Chapter 7, uremia is associated with a reduction in the protein binding of a number of drugs, primarily organic acids (1-5). Disease states can alter the binding of drugs either by a reduction in the concentration of serum proteins or by the accumulation of endogenous compounds, such as free fatty acids and bilirubin, that affect drug-protein interactions (6,7). (See Chapter 9 for a more extensive discussion of bilirubin and changes in protein binding.) The in vitro studies reported here were performed to determine which mechanism is of primary importance for the binding defect in uremia. In addition, the importance of free fatty acids in drug protein binding was investigated in patients undergoing cardiopulmonary bypass procedures and in patients with bacterial infection.

Methods

Serum was obtained on multiple occasions from 15 healthy subjects, 26 uremic patients maintained on chronic hemodialysis, 3 patients receiving a renal transplantation, 11 patients undergoing cardiopulmonary bypass procedures and 20 patients with bacterial infection. Pooled and individual sera from normal subjects and uremic patients were divided into two aliquots. One aliquot was treated with activated charcoal at pH 3.0 by the method of Chen (8). Total serum protein and albumin were measured on all sera by Auto-analyzer methods in the clinical chemistry laboratory.

Drug protein binding was determined by equilibrium dialysis (9). Sulfa-methoxazole, dicloxacillin, penicillin G, phenytoin, salicylate and digitoxin were studied in treated and untreated sera from uremic patients and normal subjects. (Dicloxacillin binding studies for patients with cystic fibrosis has been described in Chapter 7.) Only phenytoin binding was studied in sera from patients undergoing cardiopulmonary bypass procedures and those with bacterial infection. Drug was added to 2 ml aliquots of serum at final con-centrations of 40 µg per ml for sulfamethoxazole, 20 µg per ml for phenytoin and salicylate, 10 µg per ml for dicloxacillin and penicillin G and 10 ng per ml for digitoxin. The added dicloxacillin, penicillin G, phenytoin, salicylate and digitoxin contained some S^{35} or C^{14} labeled drug. Sera were dialyzed against Krebs-Ringer phosphate buffer, pH 7.4, for 48 hours at 4°C. Concentrations of drug in serum and dialysate were determined by the amount of radioactivity present. Sulfamethoxazole concentrations were measured by the Bratton and Marshall method (10). The bound fraction of drug was calculated by dividing the drug concentration in serum minus the drug concentration in dialysate by the drug concentration in serum.

The effect of serum albumin concentration on the degree of protein binding was evaluated by diluting normal serum with Krebs-Ringer phosphate buffer to lower the albumin concentration by 20, 40, 60, 80 and 90 percent.

Free fatty acids (FFA) in serum were measured by the colorimetric procedure described by Mika-Devoc, Stankovic and Boskovic (11).

Results

Studies in Uremia

Protein binding of sulfamethoxazole (SMZ) in normal and uremic pooled serum is shown in Table I.

Table I. Effect of Protein Concentration, Dialysis and Ultrafiltrates of Pooled Normal and Uremic Serum on Protein Binding of Sulfamethoxazole (SMZ)[a]

Serum	Serum Albumin gms %	Percent SMZ Protein Bound
Normal serum	5.1	65.2[b]
Uremic serum	3.9	36.0
Diluted normal serum	3.9	62.1
Dialyzed normal serum	5.0	64.8
Dialyzed uremic serum	3.9	37.1
Normal serum protein and uremic serum ultrafiltrate	5.0	64.0
Uremic serum protein and normal serum ultrafiltrate	3.8	35.3

[a] Data from reference 12
[b] Values are average of duplicate samples

The protein binding of SMZ was markedly reduced in uremic serum and significantly less than normal serum diluted to produce the same albumin concentration. Dialysis in continuously running hemodialysis bath fluid for seven days did not correct the binding defect in uremic serum. The ultrafiltrate of normal serum did not increase SMZ binding of uremic serum proteins;

likewise, the ultrafiltrate of uremic serum did not affect the binding of normal serum proteins. However, charcoal treatment of uremic serum markedly increased the binding of sulfamethoxazole and dicloxacillin without altering their binding in normal serum (Table II).

Table II. Effect of Charcoal Treatment at pH 3.0 of Pooled Normal and Uremic Serum on Protein Binding of Sulfamethoxazole and Dicloxacillin[a]

Drug	Pooled Serum	Percent Protein Bound[b]	
		Pre-treatment	Post-treatment
Sulfamethoxazole	Normal	65.2	65.6
	Uremic	36.0	58.5
Dicloxacillin	Normal	97.0	96.9
	Uremic	89.9	96.3

[a] Data from references 12 and 13
[b] Values are average of duplicate samples

The effect of charcoal treatment at pH 3.0 on protein binding of six drugs in individual sera from six normal and eight uremic patients is shown in Table III.

Table III. Effect of Charcoal Treatment at pH 3.0 on Protein Binding of 6 Drugs in Sera from 6 Normal and 8 Uremic Patients[a]

Drug	Subjects	Percent Protein Bound[b]	
		Pre-treatment	Post-treatment
Sulfamethoxazole	Normals	65.9 ± 1.3	65.0 ± 1.0
	Uremics	41.7 ± 9.3	59.0 ± 3.4
Dicloxacillin	Normals	97.1 ± 0.3	96.9 ± 0.2
	Uremics	90.7 ± 1.6	96.3 ± 0.7
Phenytoin	Normals	93.1 ± 1.1	93.1 ± 1.1
	Uremics	84.3 ± 2.6	90.8 ± 2.4
Salicylate	Normals	96.7 ± 0.5	96.5 ± 0.8
	Uremics	86.4 ± 7.9	93.8 ± 2.4
Digitoxin	Normals	92.7 ± 0.2	92.4 ± 0.4
	Uremics	89.5 ± 2.9	90.9 ± 2.0
Penicillin G	Normals	66.2 ± 1.4	63.6 ± 2.2
	Uremics	43.6 ± 5.0	47.7 ± 6.0

[a] Data from reference 12
[b] Values are means ± standard deviation

Protein binding in uremic sera was significantly reduced (p < 0.05) for all six drugs. The fraction of drug bound to protein in normal sera was unaffected by charcoal treatment for all drugs except penicillin G where a small but significant (p < 0.05) reduction occurred. However, charcoal treatment of uremic sera markedly increased (p < 0.01) the binding of all drugs except penicillin G. The effect of charcoal treatment on the binding of sulfamethoxazole is also shown in Figure 1 by relating individual binding values to the serum albumin concentration. Uremic sera had lower albumin concentrations, but the defect in binding was much less than could be accounted for by hypoalbuminemia alone. Charcoal treatment increased SMZ binding into the normal range. Similar findings were observed with dicloxacillin, phenytoin, salicylate and digitoxin, but not with penicillin G (12).

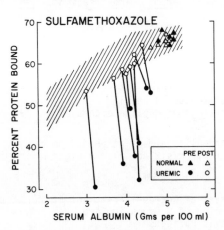

Fig. 1.   Effect of charcoal treatment on relationship between serum
          albumin concentration and protein binding of sulfamethoxazole
          in 6 normal and 8 uremic patients. The hashed lines repre-
          sent the 95 percent confidence limits for protein binding of
          sera from 4 normal subjects diluted with buffer to lower the
          albumin concentration by 20, 40 and 60 percent. (From Craig
          et al (12). Reproduced by permission of Journal of Laboratory
          and Clinical Medicine).

The addition of relatively large amounts of creatinine, urea, uric acid and phosphate to normal serum failed to produce a binding defect for sulfamethoxazole. Excessive quantities of suspected uremic toxins such as methylguanidine, guanidinosuccinic acid and guanidinoacetic acid also did not produce a binding defect.

Mean FFA concentrations in sera from 9 normals and 27 uremic patients were similar (788 ± 207 and 837 ± 770 µEq per liter respectively) except that the variation was greater in uremic patients. The protein binding of sulfamethoxazole and dicloxacillin in relation to the molar ratio of FFA to albumin is shown in Figure 2. Binding was reduced for both drugs, but the degree of binding appeared unrelated to the molar ratio of FFA to albumin. Ratios were less than 3 in all but one patient. This individual had a molar ratio of FFA to albumin of 7.0 and a marked reduction in the binding of both drugs.

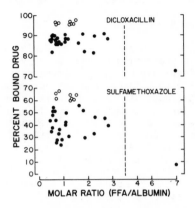

Fig. 2. Relationship between the protein binding of sulfamethoxazole and dicloxacillin and the molar ratio of FFA to albumin in sera from 9 normals (open circle) and 27 uremic patients (closed circle).

The protein binding of sulfamethoxazole and dicloxacillin in serial serum samples from 3 patients receiving a renal transplant are shown in Figure 3.

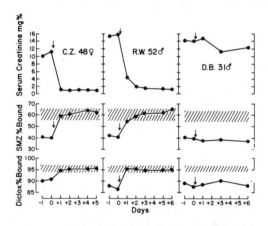

Fig. 3. Serum creatinine level and protein binding of sulfamethoxazole and dicloxacillin in sera obtained from 3 patients prior to and after renal transplantation. Day 0 is the day of transplantation; the hashed lines represent the normal binding range for observed serum albumin concentrations in each patient.

129

C.Z. and R.W. had successful living-related donor transplants. The binding defect for both drugs was rapidly corrected in these patients and paralleled the fall in serum creatinine. D.B. had an unsuccessful transplant with a cadaver kidney and the binding defect remained throughout the period of study.

Studies during Cardiopulmonary Bypass

Serial serum samples were obtained before, during and after cardiopulmonary bypass in 11 patients undergoing cardiac surgery. With the first four patients, sera were obtained only on the day of surgery; in subsequent patients additional samples were obtained one day before and after surgery. Cardiopulmonary bypass was instituted 2 to 5 hours after induction of anesthesia. The pump oxygenator was primed with one liter of Lactated Ringer's solution, one liter of 5% dextrose in 0.45% saline and two units of whole blood. A loading dose of sodium heparin (300 units per kg) was administered just prior to bypass; additional heparin was infused at rates of approximately 2000 units per hour until termination of extracorporeal circulation. Patients were maintained on bypass perfusion for 2 to 7 hours with a mean of 225 minutes. Protamine sulfate (6 mg per kg) was administered just after termination of extracorporeal circulation.

The degree of phenytoin binding, albumin concentration, FFA level and molar ratio of FFA to albumin in sera obtained from two of the 11 patients are shown in Figure 4.

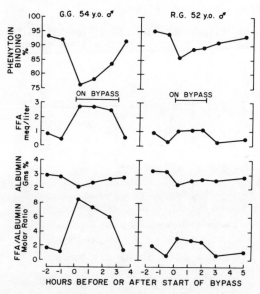

Fig. 4. Protein binding of phenytoin, FFA level, albumin concentration and molar ratio of FFA to albumin in sera from 2 patients undergoing cardiopulmonary bypass procedures. Zero hour refers to the initiation of pump perfusion.

Hemodilution occurred in both patients during pump perfusion. FFA levels were strikingly increased in patient G.G. while on cardiopulmonary bypass. This resulted in a marked increase in the molar ratio of FFA to albumin and was associated with a significant decrease in phenytoin binding. FFA levels were just slightly increased in patient R.G. resulting in only a moderate rise in the molar ratio of FFA to albumin. The defect in phenytoin binding was much less in this patient. In both patients FFA levels and phenytoin binding returned to normal shortly after termination of extracorporeal circulation. Results obtained in the remaining patients fell between these two extremes and are shown in Table IV.

Table IV. Protein Binding of Phenytoin, Albumin Concentration, Free Fatty Acid (FFA) Level and Molar Ratio of FFA to Albumin in Sera from 11 Patients Undergoing Cardiopulmonary Bypass Procedures

Serum Samples	Phenytoin Bound %	Albumin gms %	FFA mEq/L	FFA/Albumin molar ratio
Pre Bypass (11)[a]				
1 day (7)	94.2 ± 1.4[b]	3.4 ± 0.2	0.3 ± 0.1	0.5 ± 0.2
3 hours (3)	91.6 ± 3.5	3.3 ± 0.4	1.0 ± 0.3	2.0 ± 0.6
2 hours (5)	93.4 ± 2.8	3.5 ± 0.2	1.1 ± 0.1	2.0 ± 0.2
1 hour (10)	92.2 ± 1.7	3.2 ± 0.3	0.9 ± 0.4	1.9 ± 0.9
During Bypass (11)				
15-30 minutes (11)	82.3 ± 4.2	2.3 ± 0.2	1.5 ± 0.5	4.5 ± 1.7
1 hour (11)	84.0 ± 4.1	2.5 ± 0.2	1.5 ± 0.5	4.1 ± 1.3
2 hours (10)	84.4 ± 3.6	2.6 ± 0.3	1.7 ± 0.5	4.2 ± 1.2
3 hours (9)	82.6 ± 2.3	2.5 ± 0.2	1.9 ± 0.4	5.1 ± 1.1
4 hours (5)	83.9 ± 3.7	2.6 ± 0.4	1.6 ± 0.4	4.0 ± 0.9
5 hours (1)	77.9	2.5	1.6	4.2
6 hours (1)	77.5	2.8	2.0	4.7
Post Bypass (10)				
30-60 minutes (10)	90.1 ± 2.0	2.7 ± 0.4	0.7 ± 0.3	1.6 ± 0.7
1 day (7)	91.4 ± 1.9	3.1 ± 0.3	0.3 ± 0.2	0.7 ± 0.4

[a] Number of patients studied at each time period
[b] Mean values ± standard deviation

In sera obtained prior to bypass, FFA levels were higher on the day of surgery. These sera were drawn after induction of anesthesia. Pump perfusion resulted in significant hemodilution as reflected by the serum albumin concentration. This was expected since the albumin level in the pump prime was 0.8 ± 0.1 gms %. The concentration of FFA was also low in the pump prime (0.11 ± 0.06 mEq per liter); however, FFA levels significantly increased (p < 0.01) during cardiopulmonary bypass. The resulting elevation in the ratio of FFA to albumin was associated with a significant decrease (p < 0.001) in the protein binding of phenytoin throughout the period of extracorporeal circulation. The fraction of free drug increased, on the average, 2 to

131

3-fold. The degree of binding was lower than could be accounted for by hypoalbuminemia alone since the binding of normal sera diluted to similar albumin
concentrations ranged from 89.5 to 92.7 percent. All parameters returned to
normal after termination of extracorporeal circulation. As seen in Table V
the degree of protein binding of phenytoin correlated well with the magnitude
of the molar ratio of FFA to albumin.

Table V. Relationship Between the Serum Protein Binding of Phenytoin
and the Molar Ratio of FFA to Albumin in 90 Sera from 11
Patients Undergoing Cardiopulmonary Bypass Procedures

FFA/Albumin molar ratio	Number of Sera	Percent of Phenytoin Protein Bound mean	range
0 - 1	11	93.5	90.8 - 97.2
1 - 2	19	91.8	89.6 - 94.7
2 - 3	17	90.0	83.0 - 94.6
3 - 4	14	85.9	81.6 - 89.5
4 - 5	16	82.1	77.5 - 86.4
5 - 6	9	80.5	77.2 - 83.5
> 6	4	78.6	75.9 80.2

Studies in Bacterial Infection

Serial serum samples were obtained from 20 patients with documented
Gram-negative infections ranging from symptomatic urinary tract infections
to septicemia with shock. Most patients also had other underlying diseases.
The first serum sample was obtained in all patients on the first day of antimicrobial therapy. All patients were treated with an aminoglycoside antibiotic either alone or in combination with a penicillin or cephalosporin.
The protein binding of phenytoin, albumin concentration, FFA level and molar
ratio of FFA to albumin in sera obtained from these patients on day 1 and day
7 through 10 are shown in Table VI.

Table VI. Protein Binding of Phenytoin, Albumin Concentration, Free
Fatty Acid (FFA) Level and Molar Ratio of FFA to Albumin in
Sera of 20 Patients with Gram-negative Bacterial Infection

Patients	Day	Phenytoin Bound %	Albumin gms %	FFA mEq/L	FFA/Albumin molar ratio
Group A (n=9)	1	92.0 ± 1.7[a]	3.4 ± 0.8	0.5 ± 0.4	0.8 ± 0.5
	7-10	92.2 ± 0.7	ND[b]	ND	ND
Group B (n=6)	1	86.3 ± 1.6	2.9 ± 0.3	1.4 ± 0.4	3.8 ± 2.0
	7-10	91.9 ± 0.8	3.0 ± 0.3	0.4 ± 0.2	0.9 ± 0.3
Group C (n=5)	1	87.3 ± 1.9	2.6 ± 0.2	0.8 ± 0.4	2.2 ± 1.1
	7-10	87.4 ± 1.0	2.8 ± 0.4	0.6 ± 0.5	1.7 ± 1.3

[a] Mean values ± standard deviation
[b] ND = not determined

Nine patients (Group A) had normal binding of phenytoin throughout the infection. FFA levels in these patients were within the normal range. Eleven patients (Groups B and C) had decreased binding of phenytoin on the first day of antimicrobial therapy in comparison with Group A ($p < 0.05$). Five of these patients (Group C) had elevated serum bilirubin concentrations or moderate renal impairment. Serum albumin concentrations were also lower in these patients, but FFA levels were generally within the normal range. The degree of protein binding of phenytoin did not improve with treatment of the infection.

Patients in Group B also had a decreased binding of phenytoin on the first day of antimicrobial therapy. FFA levels and the molar ratio of FFA to albumin were moderately elevated in these patients. Treatment of the infection was associated with a decrease in FFA levels and an increase in the binding of phenytoin to serum proteins. The unbound fraction of drug on different days in each of the six patients is shown in Table VII. The percentage of free drug was 1.4 to 2.3 times higher on day 1 as compared to day 7 through 10, and greater than can be accounted for by hypoalbuminemia alone.

Table VII. Unbound Fraction of Phenytoin in 6 Patients with Gram-negative Infection (Group B) on Various Days after Initiation of Antimicrobial Therapy

Patient	Percentage of Free Drug				Multiple Increase in Free Drug[a]
	Day 1	Day 2	Day 4	Day 7-10	
1	15.5	11.3	9.1	6.6	2.3
2	15.1	10.3	10.0	8.0	1.9
3	14.0	10.9	10.8	9.1	1.5
4	13.7	12.3	9.9	8.3	1.6
5	12.7	11.8	12.8	8.4	1.5
6	11.2	8.8	7.3	7.9	1.4
Mean	13.7	10.9	10.0	8.1	1.7
S.D.	1.6	1.2	1.8	0.8	0.3

[a] Unbound fraction on day 1 in comparison with day 7-10

Discussion

The studies reported here on the binding defect in uremia confirm the results of other investigators that the defect in binding is greater than can be accounted for by hypoalbuminemia alone, unchanged by prolonged in vitro dialysis, and transferred in the protein but not the ultrafiltrate fraction of uremic serum (3,4,14). This has suggested that the defect in uremic sera is due to an alteration in serum proteins (4,5, 14) The ability of charcoal treatment to correct the binding defect for 5 different drugs provides evidence for the presence of a binding inhibitor in uremic serum. Charcoal treatment failed to correct the binding defect for penicillin in sera from uremic patients, but it also reduced penicillin binding in normal sera. This suggests that charcoal treatment alters the binding site for penicillin. Chen presented extensive evidence that charcoal treatment at low pH does not grossly alter albumin from a physiochemical viewpoint (8). However, he investigated the effect of charcoal treatment on protein binding with only fatty acids and a fluorescent dye.

The rapid correction of the binding defect by a successful kidney transplant provides additional support for the concept of a binding inhibitor. The inhibitor could a) occupy the binding site of certain drugs, b) change the configuration of the albumin molecule or c) both. Various low and middle molecular weight compounds known to accumulate in uremia fail to inhibit protein binding. Furthermore, these compounds are dialyzable. The inability of dialysis to correct the defect suggests that the inhibitor may be highly bound to serum proteins. Free fatty acids bind strongly to serum albumin and are known to affect drug-protein interactions (6). However, FFA levels in chronic renal failure are usually low or normal (15,16). Our data support these studies. In only one of 26 patients was a significantly elevated level of FFA observed, but that patient did have a marked defect in protein binding. Thus, while the primary binding defect in uremia is apparently not due to FFA, their elevation can compound the binding defect.

Elevated concentrations of FFA have been reported in a variety of disease states such as hyperthyroidism, diabetes mellitus and acute myocardial infarction (17-19), and it is reasonable to suspect that these diseases would be associated with a defect in drug protein binding. However, the role of FFA in drug protein binding might be more clearly examined in a clinical situation in which an elevation of FFA is acutely produced and then terminated. This situation occurs in patients undergoing cardiopulmonary bypass procedures. These patients are placed on heparin during pump perfusion, and this drug is well known to increase FFA levels through the activation of lipoprotein lipase (20). The effect of heparin is then terminated at the end of bypass by the administration of protamine sulfate. The results reported here clearly demonstrate that in vivo elevations of FFA are associated with a defect in the protein binding of phenytoin. Similar results have been reported in rats following exercise or the injection of epinephrine (21). The protein binding of other drugs may behave similarly.

Bacterial infection is another disease state reported to elevate FFA (22). Concentrations of FFA in Gram-positive infections were normal, while levels greater than 3000 µEq per liter were recorded in most Gram-negative infections. Our data does not completely support the previous study. Only 7 of 20 patients with documented Gram-negative infection had FFA concentrations greater than 1000 µEq per liter. However, none of the patients had FFA levels as high as 3000 µEq per liter.

Eleven infected patients were found to have a defect in the protein binding of phenytoin on the first day of antimicrobial therapy. Five of these patients had renal impairment or an elevated bilirubin concentration that may have contributed to the decrease in protein binding. In the remaining 6 patients the binding defect was associated with a modest rise in the concentration of FFA. Both binding and FFA levels returned to normal with successful treatment of the infection. FFA levels were normal in all 9 patients with normal binding during the acute phase of infection. These data

134

suggest that some but not all patients with Gram-negative infections have elevated FFA concentrations resulting in a defect in protein binding. There was, however, no clear correlation between the presence of a binding defect and the severity of the infection.

Summary

Chronic uremia, Gram-negative bacterial infection and cardiopulmonary bypass are associated with a defect in the serum protein binding of certain drugs. In two of these conditions (infection and cardiopulmonary bypass) the binding defect was associated with elevated FFA concentrations and correlated well with the magnitude of the molar ratio of FFA to albumin. FFA were not the cause of the binding defect in uremia. However, correction of the binding defect by treatment with activated charcoal at low pH and by a successful kidney transplant suggest that uremia is associated with the accumulation of some other endogenous binding inhibitor. Further studies are necessary to determine if the binding defect for certain drugs in these diseases will alter pharmacodynamic activity.

References

1. F. Andreasen. Protein binding of drugs in plasma from patients with acute renal failure. Acta Pharmacol. Toxicol. 32: 417-429 (1973).
2. W. A. Craig, P. G. Welling, J. P. Wagnild and C. M. Kunin. Reduced protein binding of antimicrobial agents in serum of patients with impaired renal function. IN G. K. Daikos (ed.), Progress in Chemotherapy, Hellenic Society of Chemotherapy, Athens, Greece, 1974, pp. 722-725.
3. M. M. Reidenberg and M. Affrime. Influence of disease on binding of drugs to plasma proteins. Ann. N.Y. Acad. Sci. 226: 115-126 (1973).
4. M. M. Reidenberg, I. Odar-Cederlöf, C. von Bahr, O. Borgå and F. Sjöqvist. Protein binding of diphenylhydantoin and desmethylimipramine in plasma from patients with poor renal function. N. Engl. J. Med. 285: 264-267 (1971).
5. D. W. Shoeman and D. L. Azarnoff. The alteration of plasma proteins in uremia as reflected in their ability to bind digitoxin and diphenyl-hydantoin. Pharmacology 7: 169-177 (1972).
6. D. Rudman, T. J. Bixler II, and A. E. Del Rio. Effect of free fatty acids on binding of drugs by bovine serum albumin, by human serum albumin and by rabbit serum. J. Pharmacol. Exp. Ther. 176: 261-272 (1971).
7. A. Rane, P. K. M. Lunde, B. Jalling, S. J. Yaffe and F. Sjöqvist. Plasma protein binding of diphenylhydantoin in normal and hyperbilirubinemic infants. J. Pediatr. 78: 877-882 (1971).
8. R. F. Chen. Removal of fatty acids from serum albumin by charcoal treatment. J. Biol. Chem. 242: 173-181 (1967).
9. C. M. Kunin. Clinical pharmacology of the new penicillins. I. Importance of serum protein binding in determining antimicrobial activity and concentration in serum. Clin. Pharmacol. Ther. 7: 166-179 (1966).
10. A. C. Bratton and E. K. Marshall. A new coupling component for sulfanilamide determination. J. Biol. Chem. 128: 537-550 (1939).
11. D. Mikac-Devic, H. Stankovic and K. Boskovic. A method for determination of free fatty acids in serum. Clin. Chim. Acta 45: 55-59 (1973).
12. W. A. Craig, M. A. Evenson, K. P. Sarver and J. P. Wagnild. Correction of protein binding defect in uremic sera by charcoal treatment. J. Lab.

Clin. Med. <u>87</u>: 637-647 (1976).

13. W. A. Craig. Further studies on the protein binding inhibitor of anti-microbials in uremic sera. In J. D. Williams and A. M. Geddes (eds.), Chemotherapy, Vol. 4, Pharmacology of Antibiotics, Plenum, New York, 1976, pp. 79-83.

14. D. S. Campion. Decreased drug binding by serum albumin during renal failure. Toxicol. Appl. Pharmacol. <u>25</u>: 391-397 (1973).

15. M. S. Losowsky and D. M. Kenward. Lipid metabolism in acute and chronic renal failure. J. Lab. Clin. Med. <u>71</u>: 736-743 (1968).

16. R. A. Gutman, A. Uy, R. J. Shalhoub, A. D. Wade, J. M. B. O'Connell and L. Recant. Hypertriglyceridemia in chronic nonnephrotic renal failure. Am. J. Clin. Nutr. <u>26</u>: 165-172 (1973).

17. C. E. Rich, E. L. Bierman and I. L. Schwartz. Plasma nonesterified fatty acids in hyperthyroid states. J. Clin. Invest. <u>38</u>: 275-278 (1959).

18. J. A. Moorehouse, J. Steinberg and N. J. Rosen. Sex differences in serum free fatty acid levels in diabetic subjects. J. Clin. Endocrind. Metab. <u>23</u>: 1080-1089 (1963).

19. V. A. Kurien and M. F. Oliver. Serum free fatty acids after acute myo-cardial infarction and cerebral vascular occlusion. Lancet <u>2</u>: 122-127 (1966).

20. D. D. Rutstein, W. P. Castelli and R. J. Nickerson. Heparin and human lipid metabolism. Lancet <u>1</u>: 1003-1008 (1969).

21. R. Gugler, D. W. Shoeman and D. L. Azarnoff. Effect of in vivo eleva-tion of free fatty acids on protein binding of drugs. Pharmacology 12: 160-165 (1974).

22. J. I. Gallin, D. Kaye and W. M. O'Leary. Serum lipids in infection. N. Engl. J. Med. <u>281</u>: 1081-1086 (1969).

Chapter 9

CLINICAL IMPLICATIONS OF INTERINDIVIDUAL DIFFERENCES

IN PLASMA PROTEIN BINDING OF DRUGS AND ENDOGENOUS

SUBSTANCES

Gerhard Levy

Drugs that are extensively (> 95%) bound to plasma proteins can be subject to large interindividual differences in their free fraction in plasma. The free fraction is the ratio of concentrations of free to total (free and bound) drug. Such interindividual differences may be due to hereditary or environmental influences or they can be caused by temporary changes in physiologic status, including pregnancy and disease. It is important therefore to consider the effect of plasma protein binding on the distribution, elimination, and pharmacologic activity of drugs. A number of endogenous substances are also extensively bound to plasma proteins and should therefore be considered in the same context. Consequently, this presentation will be focused primarily on one example of each: the coumarin anticoagulant warfarin and the potentially neurotoxic heme pigment bilirubin.

Studies in rats and in man have revealed large interindividual differences in the biologic half-life and total body clearance of warfarin. Fig. 1

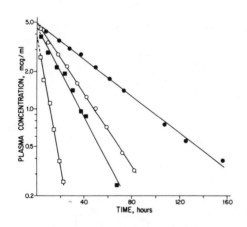

Fig. 1. Concentration of warfarin in plasma of four rats as a function of time after intravenous injection of 0.6 mg/kg.

shows how pronounced these differences can be in a group of normal adult male Sprague-Dawley rats; the half-life ranged from 5.9 to 41.3 hours in one of our investigations (1). We also observed differences of similar

137

magnitude in the serum protein binding of warfarin (2); these differences were found consistently and are multimodal in character (Fig. 2).

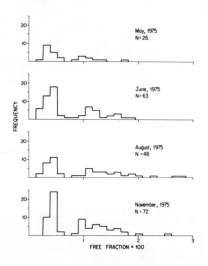

Fig. 2. Frequency distribution of free fraction of warfarin in the serum of four groups of adult male Sprague-Dawley rats.

Based on the assumptions that a) the kinetics of elimination are apparent first-order, b) the driving force of the rate-limiting step of each elimination process is the concentration of free drug, c) elimination rate is not limited or measurably influenced by organ perfusion rate, and d) the free fraction of drug in plasma is essentially constant in the concentration range of therapeutic or experimental interest, we have proposed (3) that the total body clearance (CL_T) of an extensively protein bound and completely metabolized drug such as warfarin is directly proportional to its free fraction (f) in plasma or serum:

$$CL_T = CL_{int}\ f \qquad\qquad (Eq.\ 1)$$

where CL_{int} is the intrinsic clearance of the drug. The same equation is obtained as one limiting case of a relationship which was recently developed by several groups of investigators (4-6) and is discussed in Chapter 4:

$$CL_T = \frac{Q\ CL_{int}\ f}{Q + CL_{int}\ f} \qquad\qquad (Eq.\ 2)$$

where Q is the total blood flow rate through the drug metabolizing organ. It is evident that if $Q \gg CL_{int}\ f$, Eq. 2 reduces to Eq. 1. Many, perhaps most drugs are in the category where $Q \gg CL_{int}\ f$ but a number of important medicinal agents are not. These latter compounds, whose elimination rate is limited or influenced by organ perfusion rate, have been discussed by Wilkinson in Chapter 2.

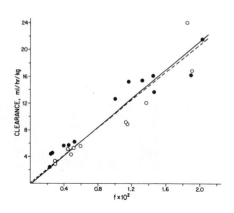

Fig. 3. Relationship
between total
plasma clearance
of warfarin and
free fraction of
drug in the serum
of individual
rats. Shown are
the results of
two studies.
Correlation
coefficient =
0.947, p < 0.001.
The stippled line
is the regression
line forced
through the
origin.

Figure 3 shows that the total clearance of warfarin in rats is indeed
linearly related to the free fraction of the drug in serum, in accordance
with Eq. 1. Thus, plasma protein binding is an important determinant of
warfarin elimination and accounted almost exclusively for the observed
differences in the total clearance of the drug. Such differences in the
total clearance of a completely metabolized drug have often been ascribed to
corresponding differences in the activity of drug metabolizing enzyme systems. The excellent linear relationship between CL_T and f found in our
study shows that enzyme activity, as reflected by CL_{int}, differed very
little between animals.

One point of obvious interest is the reason for the pronounced interindividual difference in f. Surprisingly (at least to us), this was not
due to corresponding differences in plasma albumin concentration despite the
fact that warfarin is almost exclusively bound to albumin (Fig. 4). Differences in the structure of albumin or in the plasma concentration of endogenous displacing agents are alternative possibilities and are presently being
explored.

A pathologic condition which causes an increase in f is unconjugated
hyperbilirubinemia. As will be shown subsequently in this chapter, bilirubin is very extensively bound to plasma proteins. We have found that
the free fraction of the coumarin anticoagulant dicumarol (at a concentration
of about 10 mg/L) is increased about two-fold by bilirubin, 100 mg/L (7).
Using pairs of jaundiced and non-jaundiced littermate Gunn rats, we found
that the apparent volume of distribution, the apparent first-order elimination rate constant, and the total clearance of bilirubin were substantially
increased in the hyperbilirubinemic animals (Table I). On the other hand,
the equi-effective anticoagulant concentration (represented by C_{max}, the
intercept on the concentration axis upon extrapolation to zero rate of the
linear portion of a plot of relative synthesis rate of prothrombin complex
activity versus log plasma dicumarol concentration) was decreased in hyperbilirubinemia (Table I) since the intensity of anticoagulant effect is a
function of the concentration of free rather than total drug in plasma.

139

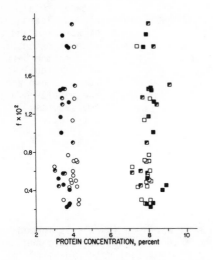

Fig. 4.   Relationship between the free
fraction of warfarin and the
concentrations of albumin
(circles) and total protein
(squares) in the serum of
individual rats. Shown are
the results of three studies.

Table I. Kinetics of Elimination and Anticoagulant Effect of
Dicumarol in Jaundiced and Non-Jaundiced Gunn Rats

	Jaundiced[a]	Non-Jaundiced	Ratio J:N-J
Apparent Volume of Distribution, L/kg	0.136 ± 0.042^{b}	0.103 ± 0.027^{c}	1.33 ± 0.25
Elimination Rate Constant, hr^{-1}	0.0743 ± 0.0156	0.0507 ± 0.0121^{c}	1.55 ± 0.55
Total Clearance, L/(hr · kg) x 100	1.03 ± 0.45	0.536 ± 0.255^{c}	2.06 ± 0.92
C_{max}, mcg/L	16.0 ± 5.4	24.0 ± 9.3^{c}	0.619 ± 0.139

[a] Plasma bilirubin concentration 6.92 ± 2.22 mg/100 ml. The bilirubin
concentration in the plasma of the non-jaundiced littermates was ≤ 0.3
mg/100 ml.

[b] Mean $\pm$ S.D., n = 11 except for C_{max} where n = 9.

[c] Significantly different from jaundiced littermates (p < 0.01).

140

To determine if the relationship between total clearance and free
fraction of warfarin in serum observed in rats occurs also in man, we
measured the steady-state concentration and free fraction of warfarin in the
serum of 31 patients with cardiovascular disease who were receiving fixed
daily doses of warfarin as part of their medication regimen (8).   There
were pronounced interindividual differences in the serum free fraction of
warfarin, though not as large as in rats (Fig. 5).   As in rats, there was no

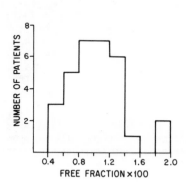

Fig. 5.   Frequency distribution of serum
protein binding of
warfarin in 31
patients with
cardiovascular
disease (8).
(Reproduced by
permission of the
publisher).

apparent relationship between free fraction value and the concentrations of
albumin or total protein in serum (Fig. 6).   Most important, we found a
highly statistically significant positive correlation between the total

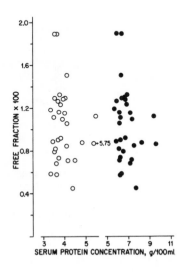

Fig. 6.   Relationship between free
fraction of warfarin and concentrations of albumin (O)
and total protein (●) in the
serum of 31 patients (8).
(Reproduced by permission of
the publisher).

clearance of warfarin and the free fraction of the drug in serum (Fig. 7).

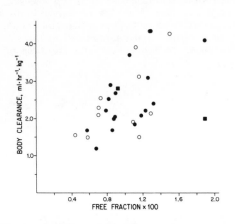

Fig. 7. Relationship between the estimated total clearance and the free fraction of warfarin in the serum of 31 patients. O, smokers and patients taking barbiturates; ● patients who are non-smokers or who smoke less than 5 cigarettes or cigars per day and who are not taking barbiturates; ■ , patients taking chloral hydrate. Correlation without the two patients taking chloral hydrate: r = 0.641, p < 0.001. From reference 8; reproduced by permission of the publisher.

Thus, protein binding is a major determinant of warfarin elimination in patients under clinical conditions.

Considering the significant role of protein binding in warfarin elimination, it became important to determine the intrasubject variation in the free fraction of warfarin in serum. As a necessary first step, one has to establish the reproducibility of the method for the determination of f. Fig. 8 is a plot of f values for serum samples from 23 patients against f

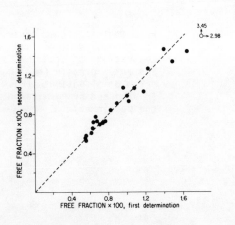

Fig. 8. Correlation between the results of two separate determinations of the free fraction values of warfarin in the serum of 23 patients. The two determinations were made on the same serum samples. The stippled line indicates perfect correlation. Correlation coefficient 0.991, p < 0.001.

values for the same samples determined a second time on another day. The absolute difference between the pairs of values was only 6 ± 5 percent

142

(mean ± S.D.), an excellent reproducibility considering the fact that this drug is very extensively bound (≈ 99 percent). The absolute difference in percent bound values was therefore only about 0.06 percent on the average for duplicate determinations. For the study of intrasubject variations in f, we were able to obtain a second serum sample from 23 of the 31 patients in our original study (9). The time interval between the two studies was 3.4 to 5.7 months and the drug dosage regimen for the patients had not been changed significantly. It was found that the f values in the first and second study were very significantly (< 0.001) correlated (Fig. 9); the

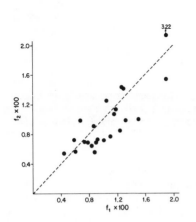

Fig. 9. Relationship between protein binding of warfarin in the serum of 23 patients on two days, 3.4 to 5.7 months apart. Plotted are the free fraction values obtained in the first clinical study (f_1) against those obtained in the second clinical study (f_2). The stippled line indicates perfect correlation. Correlation coefficient 0.740, $p < 0.001$.

average absolute change in f values was 25.5 ± 15.6 percent. Some of this difference is probably related to the fluctuating concentrations of concomitantly administered drugs capable of competing with warfarin for plasma protein binding sites. Despite this, it is evident that f was relatively constant in any one patient under the conditions of our investigation.

Since many serum protein binding studies are done with serum obtained from healthy young subjects, we determined f values for warfarin in serum of 18 prisoners, a segment of our population which is strongly represented among normal subjects used in pharmacokinetic research. As is evident in Fig. 10, the f values in these subjects were similar to those in the patients, but much more narrowly distributed. It is advisable therefore to characterize the protein binding characteristics of drugs in serum or plasma obtained not only from normal subjects but also from different types of patients.

The relationship between total clearance and free fraction in serum described here with respect to warfarin is also demonstrable with other drugs and endogenous substances. Gugler et al. (10) have recently determined the steady-state concentrations of free and total phenytoin and the total clearance of this drug in normal subjects and in patients with nephrotic syndrome.

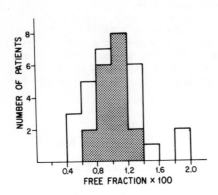

Fig. 10. Comparison of the frequency distribution of the free fraction of warfarin in the serum of 31 patients with cardiovascular disease (open bars) and 18 healthy adult volunteers (shaded bars).

The patients were hypoalbuminemic ($\leq$ 3% albumin) but showed no evidence of impaired liver function. The average f value for phenytoin was 0.10 in normal subjects and 0.19 in patients. The steady-state concentration of total (free and bound) phenytoin was considerably lower and the total clearance was appreciably higher in the hypoalbuminemic patients but the concentration of free phenytoin in plasma was similar in both groups (Table II).

Table II. Phenytoin Kinetics in Normal and Hypoalbuminemic Adult Human Subjects[a]

	Normal Subjects (n = 6)	Hypoalbuminemic Subjects[b] (n = 6)
Steady-state concentration of total drug in plasma[c], µg/ml	6.8 ± 0.6	2.9 ± 0.6
Total clearance, L/kg · hr	0.022 ± 0.006	0.048 ± 0.019
Steady-state concentration of free drug in plasma[c], µg/ml	0.69 ± 0.05	0.59 ± 0.06

[a] From Gugler et al. (10).

[b] Less than 3 g albumin/100 ml.

[c] 300 mg/day for 14 days.

Using Eq. 1 to calculate CL_{int}, one finds that the intrinsic clearance of phenytoin was practically the same in both groups (Table III). A similar

144

Table III. Intrinsic Clearance of Phenytoin by
Normal and Hypoalbuminemic Subjects[a]

	$\dfrac{CL_T/f = CL_{int}}{}$
Normal subjects	0.022 : 0.101 = 0.22 L/(kg · hr)
Hypoalbuminemic subjects	0.048 : 0.192 = 0.25 L/(kg · hr)

[a] Calculated from data of Gugler et al. (10).

finding for phenytoin in patients with acute viral hepatitis is described in Chapter 4; changes in free fraction were observed but there was no significant change in the intrinsic clearance of the drug. Thus, differences in protein binding rather than in microsomal enzyme activity account for the observed differences in steady state concentrations of total drug and in the total body clearance. This is of particular interest since the average f of phenytoin is an order of magnitude larger than that of warfarin. On the other hand, one of the assumptions upon which Eq. 1 is based, namely that the elimination kinetics of the drug are apparent first-order, does not apply to phenytoin in the high range of therapeutic drug concentrations. Equation 1 is probably applicable to the data obtained in the Gugler study, at least as a reasonable approximation.

One of the technically most challenging and interesting pharmacokinetic investigations in our experience has been the study of the effect of plasma protein binding on the elimination kinetics of bilirubin. This endogenous pigment is usually more than 99.9 percent protein bound in rat plasma at concentrations up to about 20 mg/100 ml (11). The commonly occurring physiologic jaundice of infancy is due to accumulation of bilirubin caused by the immaturity of conjugation processes in the neonate. If not adequately controlled, it can cause irreversible and often fatal brain damage (kernicterus). We have found that the total clearance of bilirubin in rats is linearly related to its free fraction in plasma (Fig. 11) and that rats as well as newborn human infants exhibit pronounced interindividual differences in f values (11,12).

Experimental hyperbilirubinemia can be produced in rats by intravenous infusion of bilirubin at a constant rate (13). Rapid intravenous injection of sodium salicylate, a strong displacer of bilirubin from protein binding sites, causes an abrupt and pronounced decrease of total bilirubin concentrations in plasma but the concentration of free bilirubin is not affected (Fig. 12). This is perhaps the most striking demonstration of the applicability of equation 1 and of the fact that the elimination rate of bilirubin is proportional to the concentration of free rather than total pigment in plasma. We have encountered some cases of bilirubin intoxication during these studies, even in control animals that received bilirubin infusions but no drugs. In these cases, the concentration of total as well as free bilirubin in plasma did not remain at a plateau but started to increase shortly

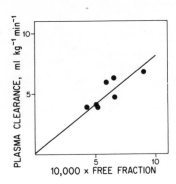

Fig. 11. Relationship between the total plasma clearance of bilirubin and the fraction of free bilirubin in the plasma of individual rats. Correlation coefficient = 0.82, p < 0.02.

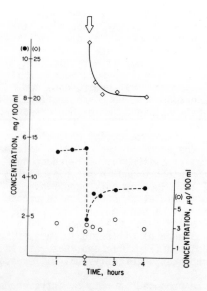

Fig. 12. Time course of total bilirubin (●), free bilirubin (○) and salicylic acid (◇) concentrations in plasma of a rat infused with bilirubin at a rate of 0.32 mg/kg/min. Note the three different concentration scales. The arrow indicates the time of injection of 67 mg/kg salicylic acid. From this time on, the rat was infused with additional salicylic acid at a rate of 0.148 mg/kg/min.

before signs and symptoms of intoxication became evident. Moreover, the free fraction of bilirubin increased considerably above that observed in vitro in plasma from normal rats at similar concentrations of total bilirubin. It appears therefore that the intoxication was associated with and likely to have been caused by two abnormalities, both referable to impaired liver function: a decrease in intrinsic clearance and a decrease in plasma protein binding, the latter perhaps due to accumulation of endogenous displacing agents.

From a clinical point of view, it is important to keep in mind the possibility that an increase in the free fraction of a drug in plasma may be caused by a pathologic condition which also reduces the intrinsic clearance of the drug. Hypoalbuminemia is frequently associated with liver disease (14). Thus, as discussed also in Chapter 4, both f and CL_{int} in equation 1 may be altered. An increase in f may be due not only to the lower concentration of albumin but may also be caused by increased formation or decreased metabolic clearance of endogenous displacing agents. An increase of f in renal disease is also only partly due to hypoalbuminemia since there occurs accumulation of certain endogenous displacing agents in the plasma.

Finally, the effect of plasma protein binding on the intensity and duration of pharmacologic effects must be considered. It has been assumed generally that the intensity of pharmacologic effects of drugs is a function of their free rather than total concentration. There is increasing evidence that this is, in fact, the case (5-17). For example, we have found that the coefficient of variation of equi-effective plasma concentrations of total warfarin in rats is much larger than that for free warfarin (18), as shown in Figure 13. It has been found that the incidence of adverse reactions to

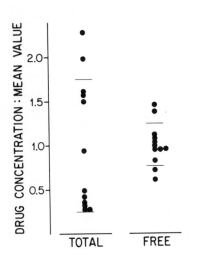

Fig. 13. Relative concentrations of total and free warfarin in plasma of individual rats required to decrease the synthesis rate of prothrombin complex activity to one-half of normal after injection of S(-)-warfarin, 0.6 mg/kg. The horizontal bars indicate ± the coefficient of variation. From reference 18; reproduced by permission of the publisher.

certain drugs increases with a decrease in the concentration of albumin in plasma or serum (19,20). This is shown for phenytoin in Table IV. Some have suggested that this is due to the decreased plasma protein binding of the drug while others have pointed out that hypoalbuminemia should not affect the steady-state concentration of free drug and have suggested that hypoalbuminemia may have been a consequence of a pathologic state which affects drug biotransformation, particularly liver disease. In fact, both suggestions are viable as will be shown here.

147

Table IV. Relationship between Adverse Reactions to
Phenytoin and Serum Albumin Concentrations[a]

Serum Albumin Conc. g/100 ml	Adverse Reactions %
< 2.5	13.3
2.5 - 2.9	10.3
3.0 - 3.4	6.7
3.5 - 3.9	5.0
$\geq$ 4.0	1.0

[a] From reference 19.

Let it be assumed that f is essentially constant over a wide concentration range, that the elimination of the drug is by apparent first-order kinetics and not affected by organ perfusion rate, that the drug is distributed in the body so rapidly as to justify the use of a one-compartment pharmacokinetic model, and that the only direct perturbation of the biological system is a change in f. Under these conditions, the relationship $CL_T = CL_{int}$ f applies. CL_T is also equal to $V_d k_{app}$, where V_d is the apparent volume of distribution of total (free and bound) drug and k_{app} is the apparent first-order elimination rate constant. It is evident that an increase in f results in a corresponding increase in total clearance or $V_d k_{app}$. The quantitative effect of an increase in f on V_d is difficult to predict but it is usually much smaller than the effect on k_{app}, at least in our experience.

Figure 14 shows the effect of an increase in f from 0.01 to 0.03 on the time course of free and total drug concentrations after i.v. injection of 100 mg/kg of a drug with V_d = 0.20 L/kg and k_{app} = 0.05776 hr^{-1} (equivalent to $t_{1/2}$ = 12 hours) under conditions where a) V_d increases to 0.25 L/kg or b) V_d is unaffected. In either case, it is evident that the increase in f causes an increase in the initial concentration of free drug but also a more rapid decline so that the free concentration when f = 0.03 will eventually be lower than when f = 0.01. This means that an increase in f will cause an increase in the intensity of the initial (maximum) pharmacologic effect but that the duration of action may be increased or decreased, depending on the dose and the minimum effective concentration of free drug. For any one drug, an increase in f under the stated conditions may be expected to prolong the duration of pharmacologic activity of small doses and to shorten the duration of action of large single doses. For example, if the minimum effective concentrations of free drug in Fig. 14 is 4 mg/L, then the increase in f causes a prolongation of the effect of a 100 mg/kg dose but shortens the duration

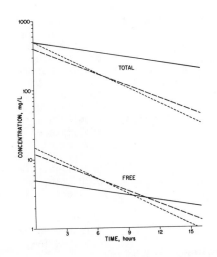

Fig. 14. Effect of a change in free fraction in plasma (f) on the time course of total and free drug concentrations in plasma after i.v. injection of 100 mg/kg. Continuous line: V_d = 0.20 L/kg, $t_{\frac{1}{2}}$ = 12 h, and f = 0.01. Short stippled line: f increased to 0.01 and V_d unchanged; long stippled line: f increased to 0.03 and V_d increased to 0.25 L/kg. These simulations are based on the assumption that the total clearance increases proportionally with f.

of effect of a 1000 mg/kg dose.

The "average" steady state concentration of total drug in plasma ($\overline{C}_p$) is

$$\overline{C}_p = R/CL_T \qquad \text{(Eq. 3)}$$

where R is the dosing rate (21). Therefore, according to equation 1,

$$f\,\overline{C}_p = R/CL_{int} \qquad \text{(Eq. 4)}$$

which means that the "average" steady-state concentration of free drug should be unaffected by a change in f. However, f $\overline{C}_p$ is only a certain kind of average, otherwise definable as f AUC/τ, where AUC is the area under the total concentration curve during the dosing interval τ. One must also consider the effect of changes in f on the time course of drug concentrations during a dosing interval.

Figure 15 shows the time course of steady state free drug concentrations for the hypothetical drug described in Fig. 14 under conditions when f = 0.01 or 0.03 and V_d is 0.20 or 0.25 L/kg. While the "average" concentration of free drug is equal under both conditions, its maximum concentration in substantially higher when f = 0.03. Consequently, it is entirely feasible that an increase in f (such as may occur in patients with hypoalbuminemia) results in an increased incidence of adverse effects even if the intrinsic clearance of the drug is normal.

Conclusions

In conclusion, it is well to point out the following clinical pharmacokinetic implications of a decrease in the plasma protein binding of a drug,

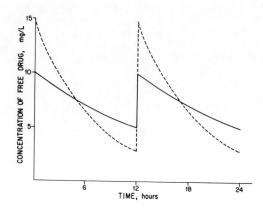

Fig. 15. Effect of a change in f on the time course of free drug concentrations in plasma at the steady state when 100 mg drug/kg are administered i.v. every 12 hours. Continuous line: V_d = 0.20 L/kg, $t_{\frac{1}{2}}$ = 12 hours, and f = 0.01. Stippled line: f increased to 0.01, V_d increased to 0.25 L/kg, and $t_{\frac{1}{2}}$ decreased therefore to 5 hours.

all else being equal:

1. The "therapeutic concentration" of total drug in plasma will be decreased. (We would not have this problem if "therapeutic concentrations: are defined and measured in terms of the free drug).

2. The time required to reach steady-state conditions by infusion or repetitive dosing at a fixed rate is decreased.

3. The fluctuation of drug concentrations between doses is increased and may necessitate a decrease in the dosing interval but with little or no change in the daily dosing rate.

Acknowledgment

The author's research described in this chapter was supported in part by grants GM 19568 and GM 20852 from the National Institute of General Medical Sciences, National Institutes of Health.

References

1. A. Yacobi and G. Levy. Comparative pharmacokinetics of coumarin anticoagulants XIV: Relationship between protein binding, distribution, and elimination kinetics of warfarin in rats. J. Pharm. Sci. 64:1660-1664 (1975).
2. J.T. Slattery, A. Yacobi, and G. Levy: Multimodal distribution of warfarin free fraction in serum of rats. To be published.
3. G. Levy and A. Yacobi. Effect of plasma protein binding on elimination of warfarin. J. Pharm. Sci. 63:805-806 (1974).
4. M. Rowland, L.Z. Benet, and G. Graham. Clearance concepts in pharmacokinetics. J. Pharmacokin. Biopharm. 1:123-126 (1973).

5. D. Perrier and M. Gibaldi. Drug clearance in multicompartment systems. Canad. J. Pharm. Sci. 9:11-13 (1974).
6. G.R. Wilkinson and D.G. Shand. A physiological approach to hepatic drug clearance. Clin. Pharmacol. Ther. 18:377-390 (1975).
7. L.B. Wingard, S. Øie, and G. Levy. Effect of bilirubin on the distribution, elimination and anticoagulant action of dicumarol in Gunn rats.
    Proc. Soc. Exp. Biol. Med. 148:397-401 (1975).
8. A. Yacobi, J.A. Udall, and G. Levy. Serum protein binding as a determinant of warfarin body clearance and anticoagulant effect in patients. Clin. Pharmacol. Ther., in press.
9. A. Yacobi, J.A. Udall, and G. Levy. Intrasubject variation of warfarin binding to protein in serum of patients with cardiovascular disease. To be published.
10. R. Gugler, D.W. Shoeman, D.H. Huffman, J.B. Cohlmia, and D.L. Azarnoff. Pharmacokinetics of drugs in patients with the nephrotic syndrome. J. Clin. Invest. 55:1182-1189 (1975).
11. S. Øie and G. Levy. Effect of plasma protein binding on elimination of bilirubin. J. Pharm. Sci. 64:1433 (1975).
12. G. Levy and S. Øie. Intersubject variation of bilirubin binding in neonatal and adult human plasma and the displacing effect of drugs. Pediat. Res. 9:284 (1975).
13. S. Øie and G. Levy. Pharmacokinetics of the bilirubin-salicylate interaction in experimental unconjugated hyperbilirubinemia. To be published.
14. H. Meindok. Diagnostic significance of hypoalbuminemia. J. Amer. Geriat. Soc. 15:1067-1071 (1967).
15. D.W. Shoeman and D.L. Azarnoff. Diphenylhydantoin potency and plasma protein binding. J. Pharmacol. Exp. Ther. 195:84-86 (1975).
16. A.H. Anton. The relationship between the binding of sulfonamides to albumin and their antibacterial efficacy. J. Pharmacol. Exp. Ther. 129:282-290 (1960).
17. H.E. Booker and B. Darcey. Serum concentrations of free diphenylhydantoin and their relationship to clinical intoxication. Epilepsia. 14:177-184 (1973).
18. A. Yacobi and G. Levy. Effect of plasma protein binding on the anticoagulant action of warfarin in rats. Res. Comm. Chem. Pathol. Pharmacol. 12:405-408 (1975).
19. The Boston Collaborative Drug Surveillance Program. Diphenylhydantoin side effects and serum albumin levels. Clin. Pharmacol. Ther. 14:529-532 (1973).
20. G.P. Lewis, W.J. Jusko, C.W. Burke, and L. Graves. Prednisone side-effects and serum-protein levels. Lancet. 2:778-780 (1971).
21. J.G. Wagner, J.I. Northam, D.C. Alway, and O.S. Carpenter. Blood levels of drug at the equilibrium state after multiple dosing. Nature. 207:1301-1302 (1965).

IV. RENAL FUNCTION

Chapter 10

PHARMACOKINETICS IN DISEASE STATES

MODIFYING RENAL FUNCTION

Peter G. Welling and William A. Craig

Introduction

The time period during which a drug stays in the body, and also the intensity and duration of the pharmacologic effect, are functions of the rate and extent of drug absorption, distribution, metabolism and excretion. Some drugs are cleared from the body predominantly in their unchanged form via the kidneys while others are partly or completely converted to metabolites, which are then also cleared from the body predominantly by the kidneys. Thus, whether a drug is cleared from the body in unchanged form, or extensively metabolized, its overall pharmacokinetic profile is partially a function of the integrity of renal function.

Under conditions of normal body function, the pharmacokinetic behavior of most drugs can be established within reasonable limits and optimal dosage regimens can be designed based on observed parameters.

When renal function is compromised, through acute or chronic renal disease, drugs eliminated predominantly through the kidneys will tend to be retained in the body and may accumulate to toxic levels with repeated dosing. If a drug is converted to metabolites, then accumulation of pharmacologically active metabolites may also lead to toxic effects. Although most drug metabolites are pharmacologically inactive, their accumulation with repeated dosing may also cause toxic reactions by displacing the parent drug from plasma protein and by inhibiting further drug metabolism (1).

The purpose of this chapter is to discuss the influence of renal failure on drug absorption, distribution, metabolism and elimination, and to describe various methods currently used to obtain satisfactory drug levels in the uremic patient.

Renal Disease

Renal failure, manifested as impaired capacity to clear material from the circulation, can result from a variety of pathological conditions. If impairment of renal function is rapid in onset and of relatively short duration, then the renal failure is described as acute (2). The primary cause of this condition may be prerenal, i.e. acute congestive heart failure or shock, intrarenal, i.e. acute tubular necrosis, or postrenal, i.e. hypercalcemia. The condition is generally reversible although complete restoration of renal function may take from six to twelve months.

Chronic renal failure is distinguished from the acute condition in that it is almost always caused by intrinsic renal disease and is characterized by slow, progressive development. Unlike the acute condition, chronic renal impairment is generally irreversible. The degree of loss of kidney functional capacity in the chronic condition is best described in terms of the 'intact nephron hypothesis' (3) in which the diseased kidney is comprised of nephrons which are essentially nonfunctional due to the pathological condition, together with normal nephrons. Progressive impairment of renal function is due to an increasing fraction of nonfunctional nephrons.

The prolonged and progressive nature of chronic renal failure is of particular concern in older patients who may require a variety of medications, both for their basic renal condition and for a variety of related or unrelated factors. The inability of these patients to excrete drugs and drug metabolites adequately, and the influence of their uremic condition on the function of other physiological systems, requires careful drug dosage adjustment to obtain adequate therapeutic blood and urine levels without increased toxicity.

Indication of Renal Function

Compounds are cleared by the kidneys by passive filtration through the glomerulus and also by active secretion into the kidney tubules. Once in the tubules of the nephron, compounds can also be passively reabsorbed back into the circulation.

The glomerular filtration rate (GFR) can be measured by any compound which is filtered at the glomerulus and not secreted or reabsorbed. Although exogenous compounds such as urea and inulin are frequently used for this purpose, the relative ease of using endogenous creatinine has made this the method of universal choice. The creatinine clearance of normal kidneys is about 110-130 ml per min; this value drops to essentially zero in severe uremia.

Combined glomerular filtration and active tubular secretion could possibly clear between 90 and 100 percent of a compound from the blood during a single pass through the kidney. Thus any compound which is effectively cleared by these combined mechanisms can be used as an indicator of effective renal blood flow (ERBF) or effective renal plasma flow (ERPF). As no endogenous compounds are cleared from the body by combined active secretion and filtration, the agent most commonly used to measure ERPF or ERBF is p-aminohippurate (PAH). In the normal individual, ERPF is about 650 ml per min. Although PAH clearance and creatinine clearance are due to different elimination mechanisms, both values appear to decline at a similar rate with progressive loss of renal function.

The radioiodine compounds ^{125}I-iothalamate ($IOT^{125}I$) and ^{131}I-o-iodohippurate ($OIH^{131}I$) have recently found considerable use as indicators of GFR and ERPF respectively (4). The main advantage of their use is the relative ease and accuracy of monitoring radioactivity compared to the chemical assays associated with conventional indicators of renal function. Both agents are cleared in essentially unchanged form through the kidneys and their renal and serum clearances are the same. Thus renal clearances may be calculated from blood levels alone.

Most studies using single, rapid I.V. doses of OIH ^{131}I have utilized segments of blood level curves or external monitoring techniques within 2 hours of dosing (5,6). Accurate calculation of clearance values using blood level data requires that the drug has reached distribution equilibrium in the body. A recent study in our laboratories, using data from 83 patients with varying degrees of chronic renal impairment, showed that both agents obey two-compartment model kinetics in the body and the terminal 'beta' phase is not reached until about 2 hours after dosing (7). This is clearly indicated in Figure 1. Although calculation of serum clearance requires that the distribution space of a compound is constant, this will not be the case for

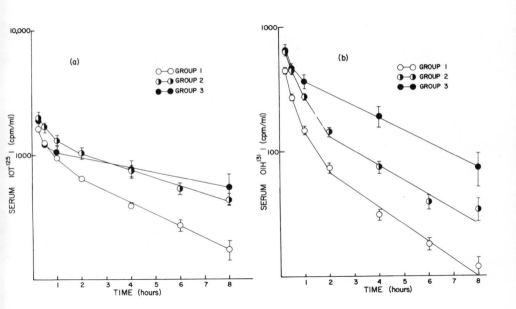

Fig. 1. Average serum levels of IOT^{125}I [a] and OIH^{131}I [b] after rapid I.V. doses. IOT^{125}I data are normalized to a dose of 2.5 x 10^7 cpm and OIH^{131}I data are normalized to a dose of 1.2 x 10^7 cpm of radioactivity. Bars indicate ± one standard error. Data from 53 patients with normal renal function—O—, 21 moderately uremic patients —◑—, and 9 severely uremic patients—●—(7). Reproduced with permission of the publisher.

either agent during the 2-hour post-dosing period when there is continuous net transfer from serum to other tissues, and serious errors may result in clearance calculations from these types of data.

Linear regressions of serum clearances of IOT ^{125}I and OIH ^{131}I, obtained during the 6- to 8-hour post-dosing period, against creatinine clearance in this study are given in Figure 2. The good correlation obtained with OIH ^{131}I reflects the decline in renal tubular secretion or ERPF, associated with general renal function impairment.

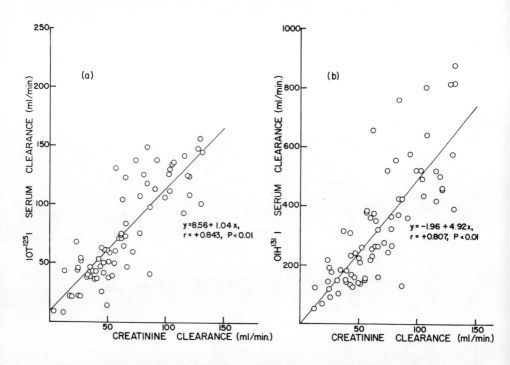

Fig. 2. Linear regressions of IOT^{125}I [a] [n = 72] and OIH^{131}I [b] [n = 74] serum clearances against creatinine clearance (7). Reproduced with permission of the publisher.

As renal function declines, the circulating concentration of endogenous substances usually cleared by the kidneys will increase. Two such substances are blood urea nitrogen (BUN) and serum creatinine. Both of these are used as indicators of renal function and both have their associated advantages and problems. The principal advantage of their use is that urine collection is not required. The main disadvantages are that BUN may be influenced by protein intake and catabolism, liver function, urine flow rate and various diseased states (2) while levels of circulating creatinine may be influenced by muscle mass, age, and sex (8,9). Further problems associated with the use of circulating levels of creatinine as a measure of renal function will be discussed later.

Influence of Renal Failure on Drug Elimination

The extent to which decreased renal function influences drug elimination is a function of the percentage of circulating drug cleared through the kidney unchanged and the pharmacologic activity of its metabolites. The great preponderance of work reported in the literature deals with antimicrobial agents while relatively few studies have been carried out on other drugs. Most studies on antimicrobial agents have described relationships between changes in renal function and associated changes in the elimination characteristics of a particular drug or class of drugs and have assumed in most cases that drug metabolites have little or no pharmacologic effect. This assumption might obviously be invalid. It has been suggested that the toxic effects due to nitrofurantoin in uremic patients may be due to increased circulating levels of metabolites (10), and the possible interactions between metabolites at high circulating levels and the disposition and activity of parent drug are known in very few cases.

The relationship between the elimination half life of some antibiotics and creatinine clearance was first established by Kunin and associates (11,12). It is clear that the influence of renal impairment on a drug half life will be a direct function of the percentage of drug cleared through the kidney. If the half life of a drug, which is cleared essentially unchanged via the kidney, is plotted against endogenous creatinine clearance, the resulting curve will be a hyperbola. On the other hand, the curve obtained from a drug which is extensively metabolized would be relatively flat. Examples of these types of drugs are cefazolin (13) and minocycline (14) and the curves obtained for these two agents are shown in Figure 3. The curve for cefazolin is typical for drugs cleared from the body in unchanged form. The drug half life increases slowly until creatinine clearance falls below about 30 ml per minute. As creatinine clearance is further reduced, the drug half life is markedly increased.

The relationship between drug elimination and creatinine clearance is better expressed in terms of the overall elimination rate constant ($\ln 2/t_{\frac{1}{2}}$). This relationship was established by Dettli (15) based on the pharmacokinetic one-compartment model. In this model the overall rate constant k is the sum of the renal k_r and nonrenal k_{nr} rate constants:

$$k = k_{nr} + k_r \qquad \text{(Eq. 1)}$$

As the overall elimination rate constant is inversely related to the half-life, the relationship between this rate constant and creatinine clearance should be, and usually is, linear. Equation 1 can therefore be expressed as Equation 2 where a plot of k versus creatinine clearance is linear with a slope of b and an intercept on the Y ordinate of k_{nr}. The value of k is

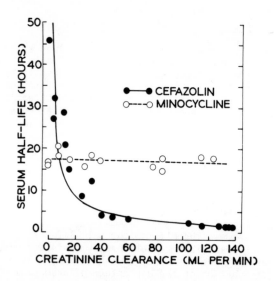

Fig. 3. Relationship between creatinine clearance and half lives of cefazolin and minocycline.

linearly related to creatinine clearance regardless of the extent of drug metabolism and provides a simple relationship between renal function and

$$k = k_{nr} + b \, CL_{CR} \qquad \text{(Eq. 2)}$$

drug elimination. A typical nomograph, of general application, which can be constructed from this type of relationship, is given in Figure 4. Equation 2 can be expressed in terms of half lives as in Equation 3 and the changes in half lives with changing creatinine clearance are given on the right hand ordinate of the figure.

$$t_{\frac{1}{2}} = \frac{0.693}{k} = \frac{0.693}{k_{nr} + b \, CL_{CR}} \qquad \text{(Eq. 3)}$$

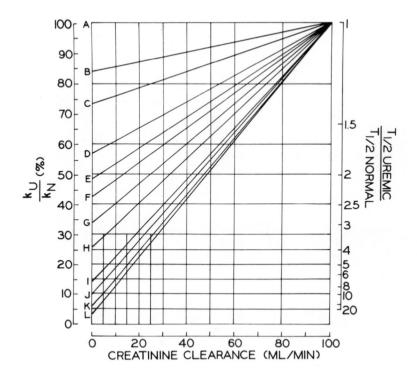

Fig. 4. Nomograph describing changes in the percent of normal
elimination rate constant [left ordinate] and the multiple
increase in elimination half life [right ordinate] with
changes in creatinine clearance. Drugs associated with
individual slopes are given in Table 1.

Each of the slopes in the figure is associated with a group of drugs
which are metabolized to a similar extent in the body. The group of drugs,
together with normal overall elimination rate constants k_N, nonrenal elimination rate constants k_{nr}, $k_{nr}/k_N(\%)$ values and literature sources are given in
Table I. Typically, drugs associated with slope A are cleared almost exclusively by metabolism and no change is observed in their elimination kinetics in renal failure. On the other hand, drugs associated with slope L are
cleared almost exclusively by the kidneys. The elimination rate constant of
these drugs is markedly influenced by renal insufficiency, with the observed
k approaching zero and the half life approaching an infinitely large value
in severe renal failure. Slopes B-K describe intermediate drug groups

161

Table I.   Reported elimination rate constants for drugs in patients
with normal renal function (k_N) and in patients with
severe renal impairment (k_{nr}), and the percent of normal
elimination in severe renal impairment ($k_{nr}/k_N\%$).

Group	Drug	$k_N(hr^{-1})$	$k_{nr}(hr^{-1})$	$k_{nr}/k_N\%$	References
A	Minocycline	0.04	0.04	100.0	14
	Rifampicin	0.25	0.25	100.0	16
	Lidocaine	0.39	0.36[a]	92.3	17
	Digitoxin	0.114[a]	0.10[a]	87.7	18
B	Doxycycline	0.037	0.031	83.8	19
	Chlortetracycline	0.12	0.095	79.2	20
C	Clindamycin	0.16	0.12	75.0	21
	Chloramphenicol	0.26	0.19	73.1	11
	Propanolol	0.22	0.16	72.8	22
	Erythromycin	0.39	0.28	71.8	23
D	Trimethoprim	0.054	0.031	57.4	24
	Isoniazid (fast)[b]	0.53	0.30	56.6	25
	Isoniazid (slow)[b]	0.23	0.13	56.5	25
E	Dicloxacillin	1.20	0.60	50.0	26
	Sulfadiazine	0.069	0.032	46.4	27
	Sulfamethoxazole	0.084	0.037	44.0	24
F	Nafcillin	1.26	0.54	42.8	28
	Chlorpropamide	0.020	0.008	40.0	29
	Lincomycin	0.15	0.06	40.0	30
G	Colistimethate	0.154	0.054	35.1	31
	Oxacillin	1.73	0.58	33.6	32
	Digoxin	0.021	0.007	33.3	33,34
H	Tetracycline	0.120	0.033	27.5	20
	Cloxacillin	1.21	0.31	25.6	35
	Oxytetracycline	0.075	0.014	18.7	36
I	Amoxicillin	0.70	0.10	14.3	37
	Methicillin	1.40	0.19	13.6	38
J	Ticarcillin	0.58	0.066	11.4	39,40
	Penicillin G	1.24	0.13	10.5	12
	Ampicillin	0.53	0.05	9.4	32,41
	Carbenicillin	0.55	0.05	9.1	42

Table I - Continued

Group	Drug	$k_N(hr^{-1})$	$k_{nr}(hr^{-1})$	$k_{nr}/k_N\%$	References
K	Cefazolin	0.32	0.02	6.2	43,44
	Cephaloridine	0.51	0.03	5.9	45,46
	Cephalothin[c]	1.20	0.06	5.0	45,47
	Gentamicin	0.30	0.015	5.0	48,49
L	Flucytosine	0.18	0.007	3.9	50,51
	Kanamycin	0.28	0.01	3.6	52
	Vancomycin	0.12	0.004	3.3	53
	Tobramycin	0.32	0.010	3.1	54,55
	Cephalexin	1.54	0.032	2.1	56

[a] $Days^{-1}$
[b] Fast and slow acetylator phenotypes
[c] k_{nr} obtained following repeated doses

depending on the k_{nr}/k_N ratios. Thus for any drug the reduction in the elimination rate constant, or increase in half life, can be predicted within reasonable limits provided k_N and k_{nr} are known.

Even when k_{nr} in severely impaired renal function is not known, it can readily be calculated from data obtained in normal subjects (23). If one assumes simple one-compartment model kinetics, then the drug elimination half life can be used to obtain the value of $k_r + k_{nr}$. In similar fashion the fraction of absorbed dose excreted unchanged in urine, f_e, is related to k_r and k_{nr} by Equation 4. From this information k_{nr} can be calculated. If

$$f_e = \frac{k_r}{k_{nr} + k_r} \qquad \text{(Eq. 4)}$$

one then assumes that the relationship between the observed elimination rate constant and creatinine clearance is linear (Eq. 2), then the overall elimination rate constant for any degree of renal impairment can be predicted using data obtained from normal subjects. In a retrospective study of 22 drugs using data from subjects with both normal and severely impaired renal function, we were able to show that the accuracy of prediction using this simplified approach was within 10 percent for 12 drugs and between 10 and 25 percent for the remainder (23). The least successful prediction was obtained with doxycycline. Although a considerable fraction of this drug is cleared by the kidneys unchanged in normal subjects, the elimination half-life is only slightly increased in renal failure. The atypical behavior of doxycycline has been explained in terms of increased excretion into the intestine followed by intraluminal chelation with decreasing renal function (57).

Elimination Rate and Serum Creatinine

Despite the susceptibility of the concentration of circulating creatinine to factors often unrelated to renal function (8,9), relationships between serum creatinine and drug elimination characteristics have frequently been described (49,52,58). The mathematical relationships between steady state creatinine concentration and drug half lives were established by Perrier and Gibaldi (59,60), as described by Equation 5 where $t_{1/2}$ is the

$$1/t_{1/2} = \frac{a \cdot K_o}{0.693} \cdot \frac{1}{C_{CR}} + \frac{k_{nr}}{0.693} \qquad \text{(Eq. 5)}$$

observed drug half life, K_o is the creatinine production rate, C_{CR} is the steady state serum creatinine concentration, and 'a' is a proportionality factor. Equation 5 may be written as Equation 6 and the relationships

$$t_{1/2} = \frac{0.693 C_{CR}}{a K_o + k_{nr} C_{CR}} \qquad \text{(Eq. 6)}$$

between half life and serum creatinine with different values of k_{nr} are shown in Figure 5. It can be seen that half life will be linearly related to serum creatinine only when k_{nr} is very small compared to k. As k_{nr} increases, the relationship rapidly becomes curvilinear and $t_{1/2}$ becomes independent of C_{CR} as $k_{nr} \rightarrow k$. Thus although a linear relationship can be assumed between half life and serum creatinine for drugs cleared unchanged through the kidneys, this is not the case for drugs which are partially or completely metabolized. Assumption of linearity in these cases could lead to large errors in dose adjustment.

Although serum creatinine levels may be relatively stable in chronic renal failure, they do not reflect acute changes in renal function. For example, it would take approximately 7 days to reach a new stable serum creatinine concentration following acute loss of renal function to 10 percent of normal (61).

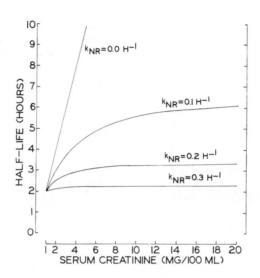

Fig. 5. Relationship between drug half life and serum creatinine
with differing values of k_{nr}. Slopes were generated
using K_0 = 50 mg hr^{-1}, $t_{1/2N}$ = 2 hr [k_N = 0.347 hr^{-1}],
k_{nr} = 0.0 hr^{-1} [a = 0.007 ml^{-1}], k_{nr} = 0.1 hr^{-1} [a = 0.005
ml^{-1}], k_{nr} = 0.2 hr^{-1} [a = 0.003 ml^{-1}], and k_{nr} = 0.3 hr^{-1}
[a = 0.001 ml^{-1}].

Influence of Renal Failure on Steady-State Drug Levels

During a repeated dose regimen, circulating levels of a drug will oscil-
late between maximum (C_{max}^{∞}) and minimum (C_{min}^{∞}) values. Although these peak
and trough levels are complex functions of drug absorption, distribution, and
elimination as well as frequency of dosing, simplified expressions can be
used if one-compartment model kinetics are assumed and if the absorption
rate constant is considered to be much faster than the elimination rate
constant, the limiting case being repeated rapid I.V. injections. With this
simplifying assumption, C_{max}^{∞} and C_{min}^{∞} are described by Equations 7 and 8
respectively where D is the maintenance dose, V is the apparent drug

$$C_{max}^{\infty} = \frac{D}{V(1 - 2^{-\varepsilon})} \qquad \text{(Eq. 7)}$$

165

$$C^\infty_{min} = \frac{D2^{-\epsilon}}{V(1 - 2^{-\epsilon})} \qquad \text{(Eq. 8)}$$

distribution volume in the body and $\epsilon = \tau/t_{1/2}$ where τ is the dosage interval (15). Similar equations when the absorption rate constant is included in the calculation are discussed in Chapter 12. The mean steady state level $\bar{C}^\infty$ is given by Equation 9 (62).

$$\bar{C}^\infty = \frac{D}{Vk\tau} = \frac{1.44D}{V\epsilon} \qquad \text{(Eq. 9)}$$

If dosage adjustments are not made for the uremic patient, then, assuming for now that V is unchanged, the appropriate $C^\infty_{max_U}$, $C^\infty_{min_U}$ and $\bar{C}^\infty_U$ values are given by Equations 10-12 where $\epsilon_U = \tau/t_{1/2U}$.

$$C^\infty_{max_U} = \frac{D}{V(1 - 2^{-\epsilon_U})} \qquad \text{(Eq. 10)}$$

$$C^\infty_{min_U} = \frac{D2^{-\epsilon_U}}{V(1 - 2^{-\epsilon_U})} \qquad \text{(Eq. 11)}$$

$$\bar{C}^\infty_U = \frac{1.44D}{V\epsilon_U} \qquad \text{(Eq. 12)}$$

The relative increases in the maximum, mean, and minimum values are then given by Equations 13-15.

$$C^\infty_{max_U}/C^\infty_{max_N} = \frac{1 - 2^{-\epsilon_N}}{1 - 2^{-\epsilon_U}} \qquad \text{(Eq. 13)}$$

$$C^\infty_{min_U}/C^\infty_{min_N} = \frac{(1 - 2^{-\epsilon_N})2^{-\epsilon_U}}{(1 - 2^{-\epsilon_U})2^{-\epsilon_N}} \qquad \text{(Eq. 14)}$$

$$\overline{C}_U^\infty / \overline{C}_N^\infty = \frac{\varepsilon_N}{\varepsilon_U} = \frac{t_{\frac{1}{2}U}}{t_{\frac{1}{2}N}} \qquad\qquad \text{(Eq. 15)}$$

The influence of renal impairment on C_{max}^∞, $\overline{C}^\infty$, and C_{min}^∞ values for drugs normally administered at different dosage intervals is shown in Figure 6. It

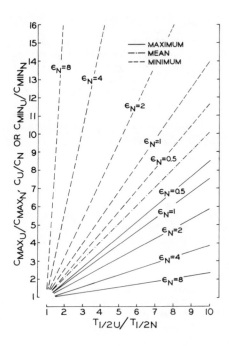

Fig. 6. Effect of increased drug half life in impaired renal function on steady state maximum, mean and minimum circulating drug levels when no dosage modification is made. Curves are generated from equations 13-15 and all values are expressed as multiples of normal values.

is evident from the figure and from Equation 15 that the relative increase in $\overline{C}^\infty$ is a simple function of the change in drug half life. The increase in C_{max}^∞ will always be less than, and the increase in C_{min}^∞ will always be greater than, the increase in $\overline{C}^\infty$. The changes in C_{max}^∞ and C_{min}^∞ values are also sensitive to the normal dosing interval/half life ratios. As the ratio is reduced, one approaches the limiting case of a constant infusion and the relative increases in maximum, mean, and minimum values will be identical.

As the ratio is increased, the relative increases in C_{max}^{∞} and C_{min}^{∞} will diverge. For example, consider a drug normally administered every fourth half life ($\varepsilon_N = 4$). If the half life of the drug is increased fourfold due to renal impairment, the $\overline{C}^{\infty}$ value will also increase to 4 times the normal value, the C_{max}^{∞} value will increase twofold, while the C_{min}^{∞} value will increase to about 15 times the normal value. If the drug were originally dosed every half life, then a fourfold increase in half life would cause $\overline{C}^{\infty}$, C_{max}^{∞} and C_{min}^{∞} values to increase 4, 3.5 and 5.4 times respectively.

Influence of Renal Failure on Drug Distribution

Most dose adjustment methods for renal impairment assume that the volume of distribution of a drug is approximately the same in patients with normal and compromised renal function. This assumption was first questioned by Gibaldi and Perrier (63,64). Using two-compartment model concepts, it was shown that a redistribution of drug in the body may occur in renal impairment resulting in concentration of drug in the central compartment at the expense of that in the tissue compartment. The argument is conceptual rather than physical in nature and is based on the complex relationships existing between the two-compartment model volume parameters V_d, V_1 and the rate constants $k_{\dot{e}l}$ and β (65).

For some drugs, however, a physical redistribution of drug has been associated with renal impairment. The distribution volume of digoxin has been reported to be reduced from an average value of 510 liters in normal subjects to between 230 and 380 liters in patients with renal disease (66). It was postulated that the reduced apparent volume may be due to a decrease in extracellular fluid volume or a decrease in binding of digoxin to tissue.

Increased apparent distribution volumes in renal failure have been associated with decreased binding to plasma proteins of several drugs, primarily organic acids (13,67-69). Some drugs for which reduced binding has been reported, and also those which are not affected, are given in Table II. The causative factor in reduced binding has not been identified. The

Table II. Plasma Protein Binding of Drugs in Uremia

Binding reduced in uremia	Binding not affected
Cefazolin	Chloramphenicol
Cephalexin	Desmethylimipramine
Cephalothin	Minocycline
Cloxacillin	Nitrofurantoin
Diazoxide	Trimethoprim
Doxycycline	
Penicillin G	
Phenytoin	
Sulfamethazine	
Sulfamethoxazole	

reduction is greater than can be accounted for by hypoalbuminemia and is not corrected by hemodialysis (70,71). (See Chapter 8 for detailed discussion on binding in uremia).

Protein Binding and Renal Elimination

The influence of reduced plasma protein binding on renal elimination will depend on the extent of reduction in protein binding, the distribution volume of free drug in the body and the mechanism(s) by which the kidney handles the drug.

For a drug partially bound to plasma proteins, the concentration of free drug in plasma C_f (µg/ml) which is in equilibrium with free drug in other body fluids, can be approximated by Equation 16 where A_T (mg) is the total

$$C_f = \frac{A_T}{V_f + 3\gamma}$$ (Eq. 16)

amount of drug in the body, V_f (liters) is the distribution volume of free drug, 3 represents plasma volume (liters) and γ is the ratio of bound to free drug concentrations in plasma.

The situation for drugs having free drug distribution volumes of 3, 12, 20 and 42 liters is described in Figure 7. It is clear that in all cases, except where V_f is equal to plasma volume, the relationship between the concentration of free drug and percent bound is curvilinear with the greatest changes occurring with highly bound drugs. A reduction in protein binding from 99 to 95 percent will result in 3.4 fold and 4.5 fold increases in free drug concentrations for drugs with a distribution volume of 42 and 12 liters respectively. On the other hand, reduction in protein binding from 55 to 50 percent will not significantly change free drug concentrations. Thus the relatively small changes in the degree of protein binding generally observed in renal impairment will not influence circulating levels of free drug unless the drug is originally bound to a considerable extent.

Changes in drug-protein binding have different effects on glomerular filtration and tubular secretion (72). Drug bound to plasma protein does not pass through the glomerular membrane whereas free drug is readily filtered. Therefore any process which significantly increases the concentration of free circulating drug is likely to increase clearance via the kidneys due to filtration. Also, as there is no change in the free drug concentration in equilibrium with bound drug during the filtration process, there is little likelihood of dissociation of the drug-protein complex and the quantity of drug filtered will be directly related to the concentration of free drug in the general circulation. An example of the combined influence of changes in protein binding and glomerular filtration on circulating drug levels in uremia is provided by sulfamethazine(69). Circulating levels of total drug are similar in uremic and normal patients. However levels of free drug are markedly increased in uremia due to both decreased protein binding and

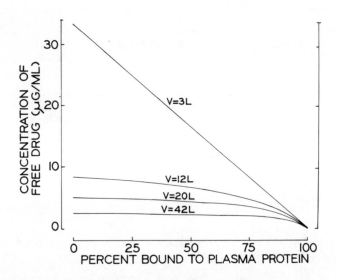

Fig. 7. Changes in concentration of free drug C_f with changes in
the percent of circulating drug bound to plasma proteins.
Curves generated from Equation 16, A_T = 100 mg.

impaired glomerular filtration. The mean ratio between renal clearance of
unbound drug and inulin clearance is the same in both uremic and normal
patients.

Changes in drug binding to plasma proteins has variable effects on
active tubular secretion. Although only free drug is secreted by the kidney
tubules (72,73) active secretion decreases the plasma concentration of free
drug causing dissociation of the drug-protein complex to yield more free drug
available for secretion. This dissociation is generally extremely rapid and
changes in drug-protein binding have little or no effect on drugs cleared by
this pathway.

Reduced protein binding might be expected to reduce renal elimination
indirectly, particularly of drugs which are extensively secreted, as a
greater proportion of drug is able to leave the confines of the plasma
volume and is therefore effectively removed from the site of elimination.

170

Concept of Whole Body Clearance

Observed changes in drug distribution volumes, either apparent or real, in patients with impaired renal function makes the concept of total body clearance or plasma clearance an attractive alternative to calculations based on elimination rate constants alone. The plasma clearance is obtained by multiplying a drug's elimination rate constant by its distribution volume and thus clearance will reflect changes in both elimination and distribution parameters.

An example of the advantage of the clearance method is provided by digoxin. Two methods have recently been described for predicting steady-state digoxin concentrations at the midpoint of the dosing interval. One method does not incorporate changes in the distribution volume of digoxin with reduced renal function (74) while the other assumes that the decrease in volume with reduced renal function follows Michaelis-Menten type kinetics (75). We obtained digoxin midpoint plasma level data from 62 patients with creatinine clearances ranging from 5.8 to 130 ml per min per 1.73 m^2 (76). We calculated midpoint digoxin levels in all patients using method 1, not taking changes in V into account, method 2, assuming that V changes in Michaelis-Menten fashion, and method 3, assuming that V changes linearly with creatinine clearance. Regressions of calculated midpoint digoxin levels on actual levels are shown in Figure 8. For perfect prediction, the slopes should have a slope of 1.0 and an intercept of zero. Figure 8A shows that if changes in volume with impaired renal function are not considered, then calculated digoxin levels will tend to underestimate the true values. Improved correlations were obtained in Figures 8B and 8C, both of which incorporate changes in V and are thus based on clearance values. The slightly better correlation in Figure 8C suggests that assumption of a linear relationship between V and creatinine clearance is reasonable for prediction purposes.

Influence of Renal Failure on Drug Absorption and Metabolism

Absorption

There is little quantitative information available on the influence of impaired renal function per se on oral or intramuscular absorption. Studies that have measured the extent or rate of absorption of sulfamethoxazole, trimethoprim (24), cloxacillin (35), and cefazolin (43) suggest no impairment of absorption mechanisms in uremia. However, as discussed below, drug metabolism may be impaired in the uremic patient and this may result in changes in the bioavailability of drugs which are extensively metabolized during their 'first-pass' through the liver after oral doses (77).

Metabolism

The influence of kidney disease on drug metabolism has been reviewed by Reidenberg (78,79). It is obvious that changes in drug metabolism will be of consequence only for drugs eliminated extensively by this process.

Oxidative drug metabolism appears to be normal in uremia while reductive pathways may be slowed. Of the synthetic metabolic pathways, glucuronide formation appears to be normal while the effect on acetylation is somewhat

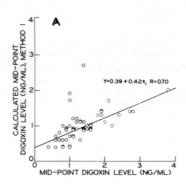

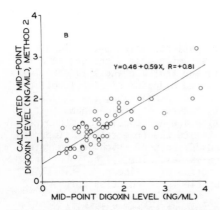

Fig. 8. Regressions of calculated steady state mid-
point digoxin serum
levels against observed
values using A: method 1
(74); B: method 2 (75);
and C: method 3 (76).

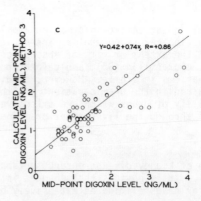

substrate specific. Sulfisoxazole and p-aminosalicylate acetylation is
slowed in uremia whereas isoniazid acetylation seems to be affected to only

a small extent.

Ester hydrolysis has been shown in some instances to be inhibited in uremia (80,81). Although hydrolysis is a relatively minor metabolic pathway, its impairment may be of consequence for such drug esters as clindamycin phosphate (82), erythromycin estolate (83), and indanyl carbenicillin (84), which have to be hydrolyzed in the body in order to release the active drug form.

Other Problems Associated with Renal Disease

Activity in Urine

The pharmacologic action of any drug which acts on the lower urinary tract, particularly antimicrobial agents used for urinary tract infections, is at least partly a function of the concentration of drug obtained in urine. The ability to maintain adequate drug concentration in urine will depend on the relationship between the kidney disease and the mechanism by which the kidney handles a particular drug. In normal kidney function, urinary concentrations of antimicrobial agents are generally far in excess of their minimum effective concentrations. Considerable reduction in urine drug concentrations can therefore be tolerated before antimicrobial activity is lost. To the writers' knowledge, the only agents which have been reported to give inadequate urine concentrations in severe renal impairment are minocycline (14), doxycycline (85), and nitrofurantoin (86).

Drug-Drug Interactions

If drug dosage is not reduced in renal impairment, increased circulating levels will increase the degree and number of toxic reactions already existing in patients with normal renal function. An example of one drug influencing the activity of another, even when dosage adjustment is made in renal failure, is provided by carbenicillin and gentamicin. These drugs are reported to have an additive or synergistic effect when given in combination (87). Although carbenicillin slowly inactivates gentamicin by conjugation between the aminoglycoside sugars and the β-lactam ring of carbenicillin, this effect is not generally observed in vivo due to the short biological half life of gentamicin. In severe renal failure, however, the gentamicin half life may be prolonged to 60 hours or greater. Co-administration of carbenicillin will then shorten the gentamicin half life necessitating more frequent dosage of gentamicin (88). A similar reaction has been observed between gentamicin and ticarcillin (89).

Dosage Modification in Renal Failure

To avoid accumulation of drug to toxic levels during repeated dosing to uremic patients, dosage adjustment may be required. Whether or not dose adjustment is necessary will depend primarily on the degree of renal impairment, the percentage of drug cleared unchanged via the kidney and the therapeutic index of the particular drug. Most penicillins and some cephalosporins have wide therapeutic indices and dose adjustment for these agents may not be essential in moderate renal impairment. Other agents like the aminoglycosides have narrow therapeutic indices and dosages of these compounds must be rigorously controlled to avoid untoward effects.

During the last five years, numerous formulas, tables, nomographs, and computer programs have been described to facilitate dosage adjustment in uremia (23,48,52,74,75,90-97). Most methods assume an absence of metabolite activity, unchanged distribution volume and plasma protein binding in uremia, and that all drug extra-renal elimination routes are unaffected by the uremic condition. The objectives of most methods have been to provide the same maximum or mean steady-state serum concentrations of drug in the uremic patient as are observed in normal renal function. That this may not be a valid exercise has been clearly pointed out by two independent groups who recently obtained high correlations between gentamicin toxicity and minimum circulating drug levels rather than maximum or mean levels (98,99).

Dosage adjustment is generally based on the type of linear relationship between drug elimination and an indicator of renal function such as creatinine clearance as in Figure 4. The degree of dose adjustment will depend on whether the investigator is trying to hold C_{max}^∞, $\overline{C}^\infty$, or C_{min}^∞ constant and will therefore depend on the relationships described in Figure 6. Owing to the simple relationship between $\overline{C}^\infty$ and k, as in Equation 9, the easiest, and probably the most practical, method of dosage adjustment uses this relationship.

On the basis of the above arguments, there appear to be three major methods of dosage schedule adjustment in renal failure.

Prolongation of Dosing Interval

In order to achieve the same $\overline{C}^\infty$ in the uremic patient as in a normal subject, the dosing interval should be increased to the same degree as the prolongation of half life. Thus from Equation 9 one obtains Equation 17

$$\tau_U = \tau_N \cdot t_{\frac{1}{2}U} / t_{\frac{1}{2}N} \qquad \text{(Eq. 17)}$$

where τ_N and τ_U are the normal and adjusted dosing intervals respectively and $t_{\frac{1}{2}N}$ and $t_{\frac{1}{2}U}$ are the appropriate drug half lives. With this method, similar C_{max}^∞ and C_{min}^∞ values will be obtained in normal and uremic patients.

Reduction of Maintenance Dose

If the maintenance dose is reduced to hold $\overline{C}^\infty$ constant while the dosing interval is held constant, then from the relationship in Equation 9 one obtains Equation 18 where D_N and D_U are the normal and adjusted maintenance

$$D_U = D_N k_U / k_N \qquad \text{(Eq. 18)}$$

174

doses respectively and k_N and k_U are the appropriate drug elimination rate constants. Thus the dose in the uremic patient is obtained simply by multiplying the usual dose by the quotient of the uremic and normal rate constants. With this method, C_{max}^∞ will be reduced, and C_{min}^∞ will be increased in the uremic patient while $\bar{C}^\infty$ will be unchanged.

Method of Kunin

With this method, originally proposed in 1966 (97), one half the usual maintenance dose is administered at a dosage interval equal to the drug half life in the uremic patient. This method tends to produce somewhat higher drug levels in the uremic patient, with C_{max}^∞ levels similar to those in normal subjects, and elevated C_{min}^∞ levels.

This method is not of universal application. This is particularly so for drugs normally dosed at intervals much longer or shorter than their half lives. For example, drugs which are usually dosed once every six to eight half lives in normal subjects will tend to be overdosed in subjects with mild uremia whereas drugs usually dosed more frequently than their half lives will tend to be underdosed in uremic patients.

Use of the Nomograph

The correct dosage schedule modifications for the three methods described above may all be obtained from the nomograph in Figure 4 by selecting the diagonal line appropriate for the particular drug type. Drugs in groups A-C are not significantly affected by renal function impairment and dose modification is generally not necessary. Drugs in groups D-H are moderately affected by renal impairment but mean steady-state serum levels would not double until creatinine clearance is reduced to 25 ml per min or less. Dose modification would not be necessary for creatinine clearances above that value. For creatinine clearances below 25 ml per min, however, dosage scheules should be modified according to Figure 4. Possible exceptions to this rule are drugs like the penicillins which are generally administered at intervals considerably longer than their half lives. Drug accumulation with repeated doses is so slight in these cases that dosage modification is unnecessary. Drugs in groups I-L are cleared predominantly in unchanged form by the kidneys. These drugs are also frequently dosed at intervals exceeding their half lives and dose adjustment is generally not necessary until creatinine clearance falls below 50 ml per min.

Consider the case of a patient with a creatinine clearance of 10 ml per min requiring repeated doses of gentamicin. The appropriate line in the nomograph is line K which indicates that this patient will have an elimination rate constant 15 percent of the normal value and an elimination half life that is 6.7 times normal. The proposed dosage adjustment alternatives are therefore to give 15 percent of the normal dose at the normal dosing interval, to give the normal dose at a dosing interval 6.7 times greater than normal or to give half the regular dose at a dosage interval 6.7 times the normal half life. Serum levels obtained from the three methods, together with the profile in a normal individual, are given in Figure 9.

It can be seen that the three methods give different steady-state drug

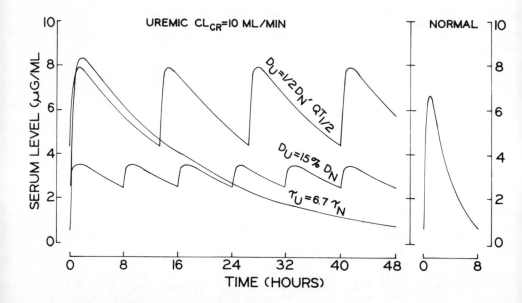

Fig. 9. Predicted steady state serum levels of gentamicin in a 70
kg normal subject and in a patient with a creatinine clearance
of 10 ml per min. D_N = 1.7 mg per kg, τ_N = 8 hr, k_N = 0.347
hr^{-1} [$t_{\frac{1}{2}N}$ = 2 hr], V_N = 14 liters and is assumed to be unchanged in renal failure. Adjusted doses and dosage intervals
for the uremic patient were obtained from Figure 4.

profiles. Reducing the dose to 15 percent the normal value yields a relatively flat profile while increasing the dosage interval gives similar maximum and minimum values to the normal subject, separated by a longer time
period. The relative advantages of these two methods will depend on the
minimum inhibitory concentration (MIC) required for the particular orga-
nism(s) and the possibility of toxic side effects. For an MIC greater than
4 µg per ml, the serum level obtained by dose reduction is of little therapeutic value. However, if the MIC were 2 µg per ml, then dose reduction would
be the method of choice. It should be noted that prolonging the dosage interval will produce inhibitory and subinhibitory concentrations for relatively long time periods. The third method of giving half the usual maintenance dose each half life yields values somewhat higher than the other
methods. This method then has the advantage of producing serum levels
greater than the MIC for more organisms and for longer periods but has the

disadvantage of potentially causing more toxic side effects in the susceptible patient. The actual method of dosage regimen adjustment is largely a matter of individual preference. Each has been used successfully but comparative studies are inconclusive (98).

Gentamicin dosage adjustment will be considered in detail in Chapter 12 and that chapter should be consulted in developing actual dosage regimens for this antibiotic. However, the above principles serve to illustrate the concept of changing doses or dosage intervals in designing dosage regimens for patients with decreased renal function.

Administration of a Loading Dose

For any drug, and for any method of continuous or discontinuous administration, the time taken for a drug level in the body to reach the steady-state is a function solely of the drug elimination half life. It follows then that, although maintenance doses in uremic patients can be adjusted to give approximately the same steady-state circulating levels as in normal subjects, the time required to reach that level in the uremic patient may be considerably prolonged. In order to obtain the steady-state level immediately, a loading dose is required. Although there is some disagreement in the literature, most investigators recommend that loading doses are not adjusted in uremia (41,48,97).

Assuming again that the rate constant for drug absorption is considerably greater than the rate constant for elimination, one can approximate the loading dose D* required to reach the steady-state peak level instantaneously by Equation 19, where D is the maintenance dose. If normal steady-state drug

$$\frac{D^*}{D} = \frac{1}{1 - 2^{-\varepsilon}}$$

(Eq. 19)

levels are obtained in the uremic patient by prolonging the dosage interval while holding D constant, the ratio D*/D obviously will not change. However, if normal steady-state levels are obtained by reducing the maintenance dose while holding the dosage interval constant, then both D and ε will decrease with decreasing renal function. As ε exists as a negative power function, the increase in D*/D will not be linear. The relationship between the reciprocal of D*/D, termed the 'dose fraction' (100) and creatinine clearance for a drug eliminated from the body entirely via the kidneys, but dosed at varying intervals in normal patients, is shown in Figure 10. The dose fraction indicates the fraction of the loading dose which must be used as the maintenance dose in order to keep the steady-state circulating drug levels equal to those from the loading dose. For example, if a drug is normally dosed every half life, ε = 1 and the dose fraction is 0.5; the maintenance dose is one-half the loading dose. If renal function becomes impaired so that creatinine clearance is 20 ml per min. the drug half life will increase fivefold, ε will reduce to 0.2, and the D/D* will equal 0.13, i.e. the maintenance dose will be about one-eighth the loading dose.

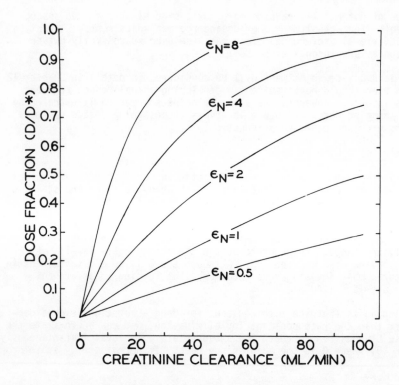

Fig. 10. Relationship between dose fraction and creatinine clearance
for a drug eliminated totally via the kidneys and dosed at
varying time intervals in normal subjects [creatinine
clearance = 100 ml per min]. Curves generated from Equation
19.

Predicted serum level curves for penicillin and gentamicin after a normal initial dose and a maintenance dose adjusted from Figure 4 for varying
degrees of renal impairment are shown in Figure 11. Penicillin G is administered as a 30-minute I.V. infusion every 4 hours while gentamicin is administered by I.M. injection every 8 hours. Details of various parameters
used are given in the figure caption. With both drugs, peak levels after a
single dose increase with decreasing renal function. This is because less
drug is cleared from the body during the absorption process. However, peak
levels in the anephric patient (curve 5) are only about 28 percent greater
than those in a normal subject (curve 1) in both cases. Curve 5 with the
single dose adjusted from Figure 4 is shown for comparison. Extremely low
levels would be obtained by this method and steady-state levels would not be
obtained before about 4 drug half lives.

Serum levels from an unchanged initial dose would continue to decrease

178

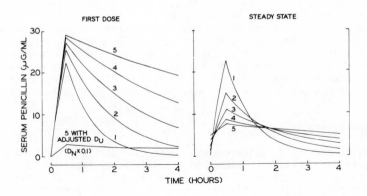

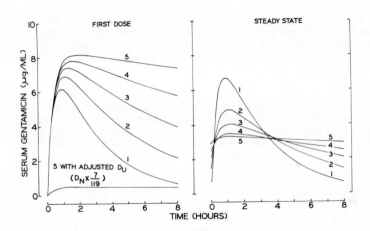

Fig. 11. Predicted serum levels of penicillin G and gentamicin in a 70
kg individual with 100% [1], 50% [2], 25% [3], 10% [4] and 0%
[5] renal function after a normal initial dose and also at the
steady state with the maintenance dose adjusted according to
Fig. 4. Penicillin G is administered as an I.V. infusion and
gentamicin as an intramuscular injection. For penicillin,
$t_{\frac{1}{2}N}$ = 33 min, V = 20 liters, τ = 4 hours, and the infusion rate
is 20 mg per min over 30 min. For gentamicin, $t_{\frac{1}{2}N}$ = 2 hours,
V = 14 liters. τ = 8 hours, D = 1.7 mg per kg with a first
order absorption rate constant of 2.5 hr^{-1}. Serum level curves
after a single dose for case 5 with D adjusted according to Fig.
4 are also shown. Curves were generated according to Wagner
(101a,b).

during about 4 drug half lives to the indicated steady-state levels. This method would provide higher drug levels during the initial stages of the dosage regimen. Although it has been suggested that these higher levels may cause toxicity, this is not supported from clinical observations (16,100). A possible exception to this rule is digoxin. Due to the narrow therapeutic index and complex pharmacodynamics of this agent, various loading dose adjustments have been proposed (102). More clinical data is needed, however, to establish the optimum loading and maintenance doses of digoxin in renal failure (103).

Dose Adjustment During Dialysis

Hemodialysis and, to a lesser extent, peritoneal dialysis are used routinely in the management of patients with severe renal impairment. The influence of dialysis on the half life of a drug is a function of blood flow through the dialysis machine, dialysate flow rate, membrane permeability and surface area, drug molecular weight, lipophilicity, protein binding, and drug distribution volume (104). Because of these many contributing variables, it is difficult to lay down general rules for the influence of dialysis on drug kinetics. Many drugs such as methicillin, oxacillin, tetracycline, and colistimethate are little influenced by dialysis whereas gentamicin, streptomycin, flucytosine, and cephalexin are cleared extremely efficiently by hemodialysis and ampicillin, penicillin G, and trimethoprim are cleared to an intermediate extent.

In addition to being readily dialysable, drugs most affected by dialysis are those cleared via the kidney and which therefore have prolonged half lives between dialyses. For most dialysable drugs, the mean half life during dialysis ranges from 4 to 8 hours (104-106). This would correspond to removal of approximately 50 percent of the drug in the body during a six-hour dialysis.

If a drug is being administered each half life to a patient with severe renal impairment, and the dosage interval is approximately equal to the period between dialyses, as with the aminoglycosides, then the amount of drug in the body will have dropped by about one-half immediately before dialysis. During dialysis the amount of drug will be reduced by one-half again so that only 25 percent of the original dose will remain at the end of dialysis. To obtain the original drug level, 75 percent of the loading dose should be given immediately following dialysis (107). If a drug is administered each half life but the dose intervals are shorter than the period between dialyses, then the 75 percent dose should be given only after a dialysis and a 50 percent dose at other times. This will cause drug levels to increase above the normal levels by no more than 15 percent immediately after dialysis and levels will return to normal within 3-4 half lives.

Further discussion of drug kinetics during dialysis is included in Chapter 11 with specific reference to procainamide and its N-acetyl metabolite.

Conclusions

Diseased states which modify renal function may influence the pharmacokinetic disposition of drugs to different extents and in a variety of ways. Decreased ability of the kidneys to clear substances from the body may increase circulating and tissue drug levels directly by prolonging the drug biological half life or indirectly through changes in protein binding and tissue distribution resulting from the pathological condition.

It is evident from these considerations, and also from the complex pharmacokinetics associated with many drugs, that there is no simple solution to drug dosage management in the uremic patient.

The methods of drug level prediction and dosage schedule adjustment described above must be regarded as guidelines only. As recently indicated by Kay and associates (108), the various nomographs and techniques currently available apply to the average, not the individual, and must always be considered in this light. For drugs with narrow indices, it is advisable to base dosage adjustments on monitored drug levels. However, this is not always possible in a practical situation.

The large volume of active research being conducted in this area, and the rapid advances being made in drug and metabolite analysis, will hopefully improve the accuracy of existing methods and facilitate more rapid drug monitoring. These objectives must be met in order to achieve optimum therapy for the renal impaired patient.

References

1. D. Perrier, J. J. Ashley, and G. Levy. Effect of product inhibition on kinetics of drug elimination. J. Pharmacokin. Biopharm., 1:231-242 (1973).
2. D. L. Guisti. Acute Renal Failure. E. T. Herfindal and J. I. Hirschman, eds. Clinical Pharmacy and Therapeutics. Williams and Wilkins, 1975, p. 80.
3. N. S. Bricker, P. F. Morrin, and S. W. Kine, Jr. The pathologic physiology of chronic bright's disease; an exposition of the "intact nephron hypothesis." Am. J. Med., 28:77-98 (1960).
4. B. J. Materson. Measurement of glomerular filtration rate. Crit. Rev. Clin. Lab. Sci., 2:1-43 (1971).
5. E. M. Sigman, C. M. Elwood, and F. Knox. The measurement of glomerular filtration rate in man with sodium iothalamate ^{131}I (Conray). J. Nuclear Med., 7:60-68 (1966).
6. M. D. Blaufox and J. P. Merrill. Simplified hippuran clearance. Measurement of renal function in man with simplified hippuran clearances. Nephron., 3:274-281 (1966).
7. P. G. Welling, A. Mosegaard, M. R. Dobrinska, and P. O. Madsen. Pharmacokinetics of ^{125}I-iothalamate and ^{131}I-o-iodohippurate in man. J. Clin. Pharmacol., 16:142-148 (1976).
8. R. W. Jelliffe. Estimation of creatinine clearance when urine cannot be collected. Lancet, 1:975-976 (1971).
9. K. Siersbaek-Nielsen, J. M. Hansen, J. Kampmann, and M. Kristensen. Rapid evaluation of creatinine clearance. Lancet, 1:1133-1134 (1971).

10. J. Sachs, T. Geer, P. Noell, and C. M. Kunin. Effect of renal function on urinary recovery of orally administered nitrofurantoin. New Engl. J. Med., 278:1032-1035 (1968).

11. C. M. Kunin, A. J. Glazko, and M. Finland. Persistence of antibiotics in blood of patients with acute renal failure. II. Chloramphenicol and its metabolic products in the blood of patients with severe renal disease or hepatic cirrhosis. J. Clin. Invest., 38:1498-1508 (1959).

12. C. M. Kunin and M. Finland. Persistence of antibiotics in blood of patients with acute renal failure. III. Penicillin, streptomycin, erythromycin, and kanamycin. J. Clin. Invest., 38:1509-1519 (1959).

13. W. A. Craig, P. G. Welling, T. C. Jackson, and C. M. Kunin. Pharmacology of cefazolin and other cephalosporins in patients with renal insufficiency. J. Infect. Dis., 128 (Suppl):S347-S353 (1973).

14. P. G. Welling, W. R. Shaw, S. J. Uman, F. L. S. Tse, and W. A. Craig. Pharmacokinetics of minocycline in renal failure. Antimicrob. Ag. Chemother., 8:532-537 (1975).

15. L. Dettli. Multiple dose elimination kinetics and drug accumulation in patients with normal and impaired renal function. G. Raspe, ed. Advances in the Biosciences, Vol. 5. Pergamon Press, NY, 1970, pp. 39-54.

16. P. Spring. Calculation of drug dosage regimens in patients with renal disease: a new nomographic method. Int. J. Clin. Pharmacol., 11:76-80 (1975).

17. P. D. Thompson, M. Rowland, and K. L. Melmon. The influence of heart failure, liver disease, and renal failure on the disposition of lidocaine in man. Am. Heart J., 82:417-421 (1971).

18. K. Rasmussen, J. Jervell, L. Storstein, and K. Gjerdrum. Digitoxin kinetics in patients with impaired renal function. Clin. Pharm. Therap., 13:6-14 (1971).

19. P. Lee, E. R. Crutch, and R. B. I. Morrison. Doxycycline: Studies in normal subjects and patients with renal failure. N. Z. Med. J., 75:355-358 (1972).

20. C. M. Kunin, S. B. Rees, J. P. Merrill, and M. Finland. Persistence of antibiotics in blood of patients with acute renal failure. I. Tetracycline and chlortetracycline. J. Clin. Invest., 38:1487-1497 (1959).

21. A. M. Joshi and R. M. Stein. Altered serum clearance of intravenously administered clindamycin phosphate in patients with uremia. J. Clin. Pharmacol., 14:140-144 (1974).

22. D. T. Lowenthal, W. A. Briggs, T. P. Gibson, H. Nelson, and W. J. Cirksena. Pharmacokinetics of oral propanolol in chronic renal disease. Clin. Pharm. Therap., 16:761-769 (1974).

23. P. G. Welling, W. A. Craig, and C. M. Kunin. Prediction of drug dosage in patients with renal failure using data derived from normal subjects. Clin. Pharm. Therap., 18:45-52 (1975).

24. P. G. Welling, W. A. Craig, G. L. Amidon, and C. M. Kunin. Pharmacokinetics of trimethoprim and sulfamethoxazole in normal subjects and in patients with renal failure. J. Infect. Dis., 128 (Suppl.):S556-S566 (1973).

25. L. Dettli and P. Spring. The modifying effects of physiological variables and disease upon pharmacokinetics--an introduction. G. T. Okita and G. H. Acheson, eds. Pharmacology and the Future of Man. Vol. 3. S. Karger, Basel, 1973, pp. 165-173.

26. S. C. Deresinski and D. A. Stevens. Clinical evaluation of parenteral dicloxacillin. Curr. Ther. Res., 18:151-162 (1975).

27. E. E. Ohnhaus and P. Spring. Elimination kinetics of sulfadiazine in patients with normal and impaired renal function. J. Pharmacokin. Biopharm., 3:171-179 (1975).

28. A. C. Kind, T. E. Tupasi, H. C. Standiford, and W. M. M. Kirby. Mechanisms responsible for plasma levels of nafcillin lower than those of oxacillin. Arch Intern. Med., 125:685-690 (1970).

29. B. Petitpierre, L. Perrin, M. Rudhardt, A. Herrera, and J. Fabre. Behaviour of chlorpropamide in renal insufficiency and under the effect of associated drug therapy. Int. J. Clin. Pharmacol., 6:120-124 (1972).

30. J. A. Reinarz and D. A. McIntosh. Lincomycin excretion in patients with normal renal function, severe azotemia, and with hemodialysis and peritoneal dialysis. G. L. Hobby, ed. Antimicrob. Ag. Chemother.-1965. Am. Soc. Microbiol., Ann Arbor, MI, 1966, pp. 232-238.

31. N. J. Goodwin and E. A. Friedman. The effects of renal impairment, peritoneal dialysis, and hemodialysis on serum sodium colistimethate levels. Ann. Int. Med., 68:984-994 (1968).

32. J. Ruedy. Effects of peritoneal dialysis on the physiological disposition of oxacillin, ampicillin, and tetracycline in patients with renal disease. Can. Med. Assoc. J., 94:257-260 (1966).

33. J. E. Doherty, W. H. Perkins, M. C. Wilson, J. Gammill, C. Dodd, and J. Sherwood. Studies with tritiated digoxin in renal failure. Am. J. Med., 37:536-544 (1964).

34. J. R. Koup, W. J. Jusko, C. M. Elwood and R. K. Kohli. Digoxin pharmacokinetics: Role of renal failure in dosage regimen design. Clin. Pharm. Therap., 18:9-21 (1975).

35. E. H. Nauta, H. Mattie, and W. R. O. Goslings. Pharmacokinetics of cloxacillin in patients on chronic intermittent haemodialysis and in healthy subjects. Chemotherapy, 19:261-271 (1973)

36. J. Fabre, E. Milek, P. Kalfopoulos, and G. Merier. The kinetics of tetracyclines in man. II. Excretion, penetration in normal and inflammatory tissues, behaviour in renal insufficiency and hemodialysis. Schweiz. Med. Wschr., 101:625-633 (1971).

37. P. L. Oe, S. Simonian, and J. Verhoef. Pharmacokinetics of the new penicillins amoxycillin and flucloxacillin in patients with terminal renal failure undergoing haemodialysis. Chemotherapy, 19:279-288 (1973).

38. R. J. Bulger, D. D. Lindholm, J. S. Murray, and W. M. M. Kirby. Effect of uremia on methicillin and oxacillin blood levels. J.A.M.A., 187:319-322 (1964).

39. M. F. Parry and H. C. Neu. Pharmacokinetics of ticarcillin in patients with abnormal renal function. B. M. J., 1:486-487 (1968).

40. R. Wise, D. S. Reeves, and A. S. Parker. Administration of ticarcillin, a new antipseudomonal antibiotic, in patients undergoing dialysis. Antimicrob. Ag. Chemother., 5:119-120 (1974).

41. W. J. Jusko, G. P. Lewis, and G. W. Schmitt. Ampicillin and hetacillin pharmacokinetics in normal and anephric subjects. Clin. Pharm. Ther., 14:90-99 (1973).

42. T. A. Hoffman, R. Cestero, and W. E. Bullock. Pharmacodynamics of carbenicillin in hepatic and renal failure. Ann. Intern. Med., 73:173-178 (1970).

43. P. G. Welling, W. A. Craig, G. L. Amidon, and C. M. Kunin. Pharmacokinetics of cefazolin in normal and uremic subjects. Clin. Pharm. Ther. 15:344-353 (1974).

44. M. E. Levison, S. P. Levison, K. Ries, and D. Kaye. Pharmacology of cefazolin in patients with normal and abnormal renal function. J. Inf. Dis., 128 (Suppl.):S354-S357 (1973).
45. C. M. Kunin and N. Atuk. Excretion of cephaloridine and cephalothin in patients with renal impairment. N. Engl. J. Med., 274:654-655 (1966).
46. J. R. Curtis and M. J. Marshall. Cephaloridine serum levels in patients on maintenance hemodialysis. Brit. Med. J. 2:149-151 (1970).
47. S. A. Kabins and S. Cohen. Cephalothin serum levels in the azotemic patient. G. L. Hobby, ed. Antimicrob. Ag. Chemother.-1964. Am. Soc. Microbiol., Ann Arbor, MI, 1965, pp. 207-214.
48. R. A. Chan, E. J. Benner, and P. D. Hoeprich. Gentamicin therapy in renal failure: a nomogram for dosage. Ann. Intern. Med., 76:773-778 (1972).
49. R. E. Cutler, A. M. Gyselynck, W. P. Fleet, and A. W. Forrey. Correlation of serum creatinine concentration and gentamicin half life. J.A.M.A., 219:1037-1041 (1972).
50. J. Schönebeck, A. Polak, M. Fernex, and H. J. Scholer. Pharmacokinetic studies on the oral antimycotic agent 5-fluorocytosine in individuals with normal and impaired kidney function. Chemotherapy, 18:321-336 (1973).
51. D. N. Wade and G. Sudlow. The kinetics of 5-fluorocytosine elimination in man. Aust. N. Z. J. Med., 2:153-158 (1972).
52. R. E. Cutler and B. M. Orme. Correlation of serum creatinine concentration and kanamycin half life. Therapeutic implications. J.A.M.A., 209:539-542 (1969).
53. D. D. Lindholm and J. S. Murray. Persistence of vancomycin in the blood during renal failure and its treatment by hemodialysis. N. Engl. J. Med., 274:1047-1051 (1966).
54. W. R. Lockwood and J. D. Bower. Tobramycin and gentamicin concentrations in the serum of normal and anephric patients. Antimicrob. Ag. Chemother., 3:125-129 (1973).
55. S. R. Westenfelder, P. G. Welling, and P.O. Madsen. Efficacy and pharmacokinetics of tobramycin in patients with chronic urinary tract infections and various degrees of renal impairment. Infection, 2:76-69 (1974).
56. R. R. Bailey, P. E. Gower, and C. H. Dash. The effect of impairment of renal function and haemodialysis on serum and urine levels of cephalexin. Postgrad. Med. J., 46 (Suppl.):60-64 (1970).
57. A. Whelton, M. Schach von Wittenau, T. M. Twomey, W. G. Walker, and J. R. Bianchine. Doxycycline pharmacokinetics in the absence of renal function. Kidney Internat., 5:365-371 (1974).
58. M. C. McHenry, T. L. Gavan, R. W. Gifford, N. A. Geurkink, R. A. van Omnen, M. A. Town, and J. G. Wagner. Gentamicin dosages for renal insufficiency. Adjustments based on endogenous creatinine clearance and serum creatinine concentration. Ann. Intern. Med., 74:192-197 (1971).
59. D. Perrier and M. Gibaldi. Serum creatinine and drug half lives in renal failure. J.A.M.A., 221:918 (1972).
60. D. Perrier and M. Gibaldi. Estimation of drug elimination in renal failure. J. Clin. Pharmacol., 13:458-462 (1973).
61. W. L. Chiou and F. H. Hsu. Pharmacokinetics of creatinine in man and its implications in the monitoring of renal function and in dosage regimen modifications in patients with renal insufficiency. J. Clin. Pharmacol., 16:427-434 (1975).

62. J. G. Wagner, J. I. Northam, C. D. Alway, and O. S. Carpenter. Blood levels of drug at the equilibrium state after multiple dosing. Nature, 207:1301-1302 (1965).

63. M. Gibaldi and D. Perrier. Drug elimination and apparent volume of distribution in multi-compartment systems. J. Pharm. Sci., 61:952-953 (1972).

64. M. Gibaldi and D. Perrier. Drug distribution and renal failure. J. Clin. Pharmacol., 12:201-204 (1972).

65. W. J. Jusko and M. Gibaldi. Effects of change in elimination on various parameters of the two-compartment open model. J. Pharm. Sci., 61:1270-1273 (1972).

66. R. H. Reuning, R. A. Sams, and R. E. Notari. Role of pharmacokinetics in drug dosage adjustment. I. Pharmacologic effect kinetics and apparent volume of distribution of digoxin. J. Clin. Pharmacol., 13:127-141 (1973).

67. W. A. Craig, P. G. Welling, J. P. Wagnild, and C. M. Kunin. Reduced protein binding of antimicrobial agents in serum of patients with impaired renal function. D. K. Darkos, ed. Progress in chemotherapy. Hellenic Society of Chemotherapy, Athens, Greece, 1974, pp. 722-725.

68. M. M. Reidenberg, I. Odar-Cederlöf, C. von Bahr, O. Borga, and F. Sjöqvist. Protein binding of diphenylhydantoin and desmethylimipramine in plasma from patients with poor renal function. N. Engl. J. Med., 285:264-267 (1971).

69. E. Fischer. Renal excretion of sulfadimidine in normal and uraemic subjects. Lancet, 2:210-212 (1972).

70. M. M. Reidenberg and M. Affrime. Influence of disease on binding of drugs to plasma proteins. Ann. N. Y. Acad. Sci., 226:115-126 (1973).

71. A. H. Anton and W. T. Corey. Plasma protein binding of sulfonamides in anephric patients. Fed. Proc., 30:629 (1971).

72. J. Koch-Weser and E. M. Sellers. Binding of drugs to serum albumin. Part 1. New Engl. J. Med., 294:311-316 (1976).

73. J. Koch-Weser and E. M. Sellers. Binding of drugs to serum albumin. Part 2. New Engl. J. Med., 294:526-530 (1976).

74. J. G. Wagner, J. D. Yates, P. W. Willis, E. Sakmar, and R. G. Stoll. Correlation of plasma levels of digoxin in cardiac patients with dose and measures of renal function. Clin. Pharm. Therap., 15:291-301 (1974).

75. W. J. Jusko, S. J. Szefler, and A. L. Goldfarb. Pharmacokinetic design of digoxin dosage regimens in relation to renal function. J. Clin. Pharmacol., 14:525-535 (1974).

76. M. Paulson and P. G. Welling, unpublished data.

77. M. Gibaldi, R. N. Boyes, and S. Feldman. Influence of first-pass effect on availability of drugs on oral administration. J. Pharm. Sci., 60:1338-1340 (1971).

78. M. M. Reidenberg. Renal function and drug action. W. B. Saunders Company, Philadelphia, 1971, pp. 19-31.

79. M. M. Reidenberg. Kidney disease and drug metabolism. Med. Clin. N. Amer., 58:1059-1062 (1974).

80. J. H. Holmes, S. Nakamoto, and K. C. Sawyer. Changes in blood composition before and after dialysis with the Kolff twin coil kidney. Trans. Amer. Soc. Artif. Intern. Organs, 4:16-23 (1958).

81. M. M. Reidenberg, M. James, and L. G. Dring. The rate of procaine hydrolysis in serum of normal subjects and diseased patients. Clin. Pharm. Therap., 13:279-284 (1972).

82. R. M. DeHaan, C. M. Metzler, D. Schellenberg, and W. D. Vandenbosch. Pharmacokinetic studies of clindamycin phosphate. J. Clin. Pharmacol., 13:190-209 (1973).

83. P. L. Tardrew, J. C. H. Mao, and D. Kenney. Antibacterial activity of 2'-esters of erythromycin. Appl. Microbiol., 18:159-165 (1969).

84. R. R. Bailey, J. B. Eastwood, and R. B. Vaughan. The pharmacokinetics of an oral form of carbenicillin in patients with renal failure. Postgrad. Med. J., 48:422-426 (1972).

85. C. E. Cox. Intravenously administered doxycycline therapy of infections of the genitourinary tract. Clin. Med., 80:30-35 (1973).

86. J. H. Felts, D. M. Hayes, J. A. Gergen, and J. F. Toole. Neural, hematologic and bacteriologic effects of nitrofurantoin in renal insufficiency. Amer. J. Med., 51:331-339 (1971).

87. V. T. Andriole. Synergy of carbenicillin and gentamicin in experimental infection with pseudomonas. J. Infect. Dis., 124:46-55 (1971).

88. L. J. Riff and G. G. Jackson. Laboratory and clinical conditions for gentamicin inactivation by carbenicillin. Arch. Intern. Med., 130: 887-891 (1972).

89. M. Davies, J. R. Morgan, and C. Arand. Interactions of carbenicillin and ticarcillin with gentamicin. Antimicrob. Ag. Chemother., 7:431-434 (1975).

90. L. Dettli, P. Spring, and S. Ryter. Multiple dose kinetics and drug dosage in patients with kidney disease. Acta. Pharmacol. Toxicol., 29 (Suppl.):211-224 (1971).

91. L. Dettli and P. Spring. The modifying effects of physiological variables and disease upon pharmacokinetics - an introduction. Pharmacology and the future of man. Proc. 5th Int. Congr. Pharmacology. San Francisco, 1972, Vol. 3, pp. 165-173, S. Karger, Basel, 1973.

92. G. E. Schumacher. Practical pharmacokinetic techniques for drug consultation and evaluation. II: A perspective on the renal impaired patient. Am. J. Hosp. Pharm., 30:824-830 (1973).

93. L. Dettli. Individualization of drug dosage in patients with renal disease. Med. Clin. N. Amer., 58:977-985 (1974).

94. T. N. Tozer. Nomogram for modification of dosage regimens in patients with chronic renal impairment. J. Pharmacokin. Biopharm., 2:13-28 (1974).

95. W. M. Bennett, I. Singer, C. J. Coggins. A guide to drug therapy in renal failure. J.A.M.A., 230:1544-1561 (1974).

96. G. E. Schumacher. Practical pharmacokinetic techniques for drug consultation and evaluation. IV: Gentamicin blood level versus time profiles of various dosage regimens recommended for renal impairment. Am. J. Hosp. Pharm., 32:299-308 (1975).

97. C. M. Kunin. A guide to the use of antibiotics in patients with renal disease. A table of recommended doses and factors governing serum levels. Ann. Intern. Med., 67:151-158 (1967).

98. E. L. Goodman, J. van Gelder, R. Holmes, A. R. Hull, and J. P. Sanford. Prospective comparative study of variable dosage and variable frequency regimens for administration of gentamicin. Antimicrob. Ag. Chemother., 8:434-438 (1975).

99. J. G. Dahlgreen, E. T. Anderson, and W. L. Hewitt. Gentamicin blood levels: a guide to nephrotoxicity. Antimicrob. Ag. Chemother., 8:58-62 (1975).

100. L. C. Dettli. Drug dosage in patients with renal disease. Clin. Pharm. Therap., 16:274-280 (1974).

101. J. G. Wagner. Fundamentals of clinical pharmacokinetics. Drug Intelligence Publications, Hamilton, Illinois, 1975, pp. 72(a), 144(b).

102. J. G. Wagner. Loading and maintenance doses of digoxin in patients with normal renal function and those with severely impaired renal function. J. Clin. Pharmacol., 14:329-338 (1974).

103. W. L. Chiou. Potential problem in digoxin therapy due to variation in recommended dosage regimens. J. Clin. Pharmacol., 15:272-275 (1975).

104. J. H. Knepshield, G. E. Schreiner, D. T. Lowenthal, and M. C. Gelfand. Dialysis of poisons and drugs--Annual review. Amer. Soc. Artif. Int. Organs, 19:590-632 (1973).

105. E. Iisalo and J. Forsstrom. Elimination of digoxin during maintenance haemodialysis. Ann. Clin. Res., 6:203-206 (1974).

106. A. L. Babb, R. P. Popovich, T. G. Christopher, and B. H. Scribner. The genesis of the square meter-hour hypothesis. Trans. Amer. Soc. Artif. Intern. Organs, 17:81-91 (1971).

107. M. Danish, R. Schultz, and W. J. Jusko. Pharmacokinetics of gentamicin and kanamycin during hemodialysis. Antimicrob. Ag. Chemother., 6:841-847 (1974).

108. D. Kaye, M. E. Levison, and E. D. Labovitz. The unpredictability of serum concentrations of gentamicin: Pharmacokinetics of gentamicin in patients with normal and abnormal renal function. J. Inf. Dis., 130:150-154 (1974).

Chapter 11

THE INFLUENCE OF RENAL DISEASE ON THE ELIMINATION OF

PROCAINAMIDE AND THE ACCUMULATION OF N-ACETYLPROCAINAMIDE,

AN ACTIVE METABOLITE

Thomas P. Gibson, Edward Matusik

William A. Briggs

It has now become apparent that cardiovascular disease is the leading cause of death in patients on chronic hemodialysis (1). The incidence of cardiovascular disease as manifested by severe atherosclerosis presenting as myocardial infarction is similar to that encountered in familial Type 2 hyperlipoproteinemia and many times higher than for treated hypertensive or normal individuals (2). Over one half of all deaths resulting from myocardial infarction regardless of the patient population are sudden and due to ventricular arrhythmias (3,4).

In the coronary care setting lidocaine would be the initial drug of choice for immediate therapy but its use is limited by the necessity of intravenous administration (5). For the chronic suppression or prevention of ventricular arrhythmias either procainamide or quinidine are the drugs of choice since they can be administered orally. Both have almost identical effects on the transmembrane potentials and electrical activity of cells from all parts of the mammalian heart (6,7). The decision to use either procainamide or quinidine for long term therapy in a patient with end stage renal failure would then depend upon physician preference, patient tolerance, and knowledge of the influence of renal failure upon the metabolism and disposition of the drug.

In normal individuals from 10-17% of a dose of quinidine is excreted unchanged in the urine and the rest is hydroxylated in the liver to more polar and antiarrhythmically less active compounds (8,9). Recent studies have shown that the half life ($T\frac{1}{2}$) of quinidine is not prolonged in renal disease (10) and may in fact be shorter (11) than in normals. However, it has been demonstrated that metabolites of quinidine do accumulate in such patients (10). Whether these metabolites accumulate to such an extent as to be of therapeutic or toxic importance is as yet unknown.

Quinidine is about 80% protein bound (12) in both normals and in patients with renal disease and therefore hemodialysis is of little benefit in the treatment of excessive blood levels. Whether the metabolites of quinidine are dialyzable remains to be determined.

The most troublesome aspect of quinidine usage is that from 20-30% of patients taking quinidine experience some adverse reaction of which severe thrombocytopenia and sudden death, even with doses of 1.2 grams per day, are the most distressing (13).

Because of the high incidence of adverse reactions to quinidine we have undertaken a study of the effect of renal failure and hemodialysis on the disposition and metabolism of procainamide.

Procainamide was first used clinically in 1951 (14). At that time studies indicated that 50-60% of a given dose was eliminated unchanged in the urine and the T½ in serum was about three hours (14). Since such a large amount of the drug was excreted unchanged in the urine many authors suggested (15) or found (16,17) that serum levels were elevated and the T½ prolonged in patients with some form of renal impairment. None of these reports, however, studied the metabolism of procainamide in patients requiring maintenance hemodialysis.

To determine the effect of end stage renal disease on the elimination of procainamide five subjects with normal renal function and twenty requiring hemodialysis, ten nephric and ten anephric, were given 500 mg of procainamide HCl orally (18). Patients were studied on interdialysis days. Serum concentrations of procainamide were measured by both fluorometry (19) and photometry (14) and the T½ determined by least square regression analysis of the terminal portion of the log concentration versus time curve.

Table I. Procainamide Half Life on a Nondialysis Day

Group	Dose mg/kg	T½ (Hrs) Photometry	T½ (Hrs) Fluorometry	Renal Function ml/min
Control (N=5)	6.4 ± 0.5	3.2 ± 0.3	3.5 ± 0.4[a]	119 ± 4.6
Nephric (N=10)	8.0 ± 0.5[c]	10.1 ± 1.5[b]	12.8 ± 1.8[ad]	<10
Anephric (N=10)	8.2 ± 0.5[d]	12.5 ± 1.4[b]	19.3 ± 5.0[ab]	

a = Not significant within group
b = p < 0.001 compared to control
c = p < 0.05 compared to control
d = p < 0.01 compared to control

Both methods gave essentially identical results in the normal subjects (see Table I). In the nephric subjects the T½ was significantly prolonged when compared to controls but the T½ as determined by fluorometry was greater

190

than that measured by photometry. In the anephric subjects the T½ was longer than in the nephrics especially when measured by fluorometry. Although the renal excretion of procainamide was not measured in the nephric patients, the slightly shorter T½ in this group was probably due to some renal elimination of the drug. However, the difference in the T½ as measured by fluorometry as compared to that determined by photometry was unexplained.

Since both methods of analysis, as done then, depended upon the extraction of alkalinized serum into benzene and the back extraction into 1 N HCl, it was thought possible that the recently discovered metabolite of procainamide, N-acetylprocainamide (20) might be contributing to the discrepancy. The photometric method, utilizing the Bratton-Marshall reaction, depends upon the formation of a diazonium salt with a primary amine and is specific for primary amines (21). Photometry should not be affected by N-acetylprocainamide since it is not a primary amine. The fluorometric method depends upon the unique spectral properties of a compound and may be influenced by the presence of other compounds that may fluoresce under the conditions of the assay. In both methods N-acetylprocainamide could be hydrolyzed to procainamide in the 1 N HCl.

Fig. 1.

Effects of allowing samples containing N-acetylprocainamide to stand in 1 N HCl at room temperature. Each point represents mean ± SEM of 10 samples. P, Procainamide, NAP, N-acetylprocainamide (18). Reproduced with permission of the publisher.

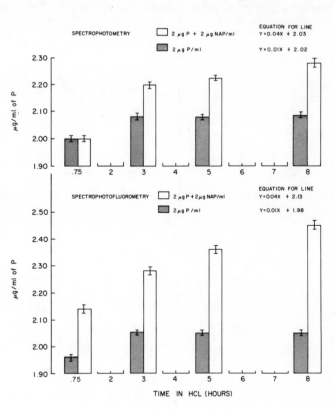

191

To determine the effect of acid hydrolysis of N-acetylprocainamide to procainamide on the measurement of serum procainamide concentration, 20 serum samples to which procainamide, 2 mcg/ml, alone was added and 20 samples to which 2 mcg/ml each of procainamide and N-acetylprocainamide were added were carried through the entire procedure. The time for all stages of the extraction was kept constant except the time the sample remained in the 1 N HCl. The two sets of 20 samples each were divided into 10 samples to be analyzed by fluorometry and 10 samples to be measured by photometry. For each time period 40 samples were analyzed. There was little change in the value of procainamide in those samples with procainamide alone by either method (Fig. 1). When both procainamide and N-acetylprocainamide were present, the value for procainamide increased with time by both methods and the rate of change as determined by the slope of the linear regression lines was essentially identical. However, when measured by fluorometry the values were greater ($p < 0.02$) than those determined by photometry. Therefore, as the sample remains in the 1 N HCl, the amine bond between the acetyl group on N-acetylprocainamide is hydrolyzed to give procainamide as a product, thereby increasing the amount of procainamide measured by either method (Fig. 2). Furthermore, it was postulated and later confirmed (22) that the emission spectrum of N-acetylprocainamide slightly overlaps that of procainamide but that the presence of the metabolite did not significantly interfere with the determination of procainamide by fluorometry if the concentration of the acid was reduced to 0.1 N, in which case no hydrolysis takes place for at least 48 hours. Also it was found that in 0.1 N HCl N-acetylprocainamide fluoresces while procainamide is selectively quenched (22). The opposite is true when the pH is raised to 11.

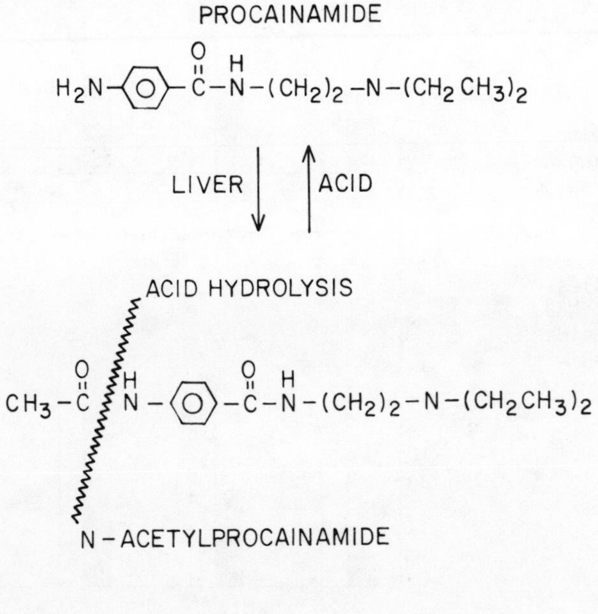

PROCAINAMIDE

$$H_2N-\bigcirc-\overset{\overset{O}{\|}}{C}-\overset{\overset{H}{}}{N}-(CH_2)_2-N-(CH_2CH_3)_2$$

LIVER $\downarrow$ $\uparrow$ ACID

ACID HYDROLYSIS

$$CH_3-\overset{\overset{O}{\|}}{C}\ \overset{\overset{H}{}}{N}-\bigcirc-\overset{\overset{O}{\|}}{C}-\overset{\overset{H}{}}{N}-(CH_2)_2-N-(CH_2CH_3)_2$$

N – ACETYLPROCAINAMIDE

Fig. 2. Hydrolysis of N-acetylprocainamide.

Procainamide has as its most common side effect the production of a
systemic lupus erythematosus like syndrome. Some 83% of asymptomatic patients
taking the drug for long periods of time will develop abnormal serological
findings (23) and some 5-20% or more will become symptomatic (24,25). Two
other drugs that may also cause this syndrome are hydralazine and INH. The
syndrome seems to develop most frequently in individuals exposed to hydralazine or INH who are genetically slow acetylators (26).

To assess the extent of acetylation of procainamide to N-acetylprocainamide we studied 14 normal subjects with normal renal function, 10 of whom
were slow acetylators of INH and 4 of whom were fast (27). All subjects were
given 6.5 mg/kg of procainamide HCl orally and the amount of unchanged procainamide and N-acetylprocainamide eliminated in the urine over 72 hours was
determined (Table II). Fast INH acetylators had a tendency to eliminate less
of the total dose as unchanged procainamide than did slow INH acetylators
(49.8% and 53.1%, respectively, p>0.4). Fast acetylators of INH eliminated
a significantly larger portion of the dose of procainamide as N-acetyl
procainamide than did slow INH acetylators (23.4% and 12.4%, respectively,
p<0.05). In addition the proportion of the total amount of the dose recovered in the urine as N-acetylprocainamide was 32% in the fast and 19% in
the slow acetylators, (p<0.01). That procainamide was a substrate for polymorphic N-acetyltransferase was suggested by these studies and subsequently
confirmed by others (28-30).

Table II. Recovery of Procainamide and N-acetylprocainamide
in Urine of Fast and Slow INH Acetylators

INH Acetylation Phenotype	% Dose Excreted		$\dfrac{NAPA}{PA + NAPA}$
	PA	NAPA	
Slow (N=10)	53.1 ± 3.6	12.4 ± 1.4	19.0 ± 2
Fast (N=4)	49.8 ± 4.0[a]	23.4 ± 3.4[b]	31.7 ± 2.8[c]

PA   = Procainamide
NAPA = N-acetylprocainamide
a   = No difference between fast and slow
b   = p < 0.05 compared to slow
c   = p < 0.01 compared to slow

Other studies have indicated that the $T\frac{1}{2}$ of intravenously administered
N-acetylprocainamide was 6.6 hours in three subjects with normal renal function (31). Eighty-seven percent of the dose was recovered unchanged in the
urine. The longer $T\frac{1}{2}$ of N-acetylprocainamide as compared to procainamide is
in part due to the fact that the renal clearance of N-acetylprocainamide is
1.2 times that of creatinine while the clearance of procainamide is at least

twice the simultaneously measured creatinine clearance (29,30). These studies indicate that N-acetylprocainamide is almost totally dependent upon renal function for elimination and is not further metabolized. Therefore it would be expected to accumulate as renal function decreases.

Four normal subjects and three patients requiring maintenance hemo-dialysis were given 6.5 mg/kg of procainamide HCl orally and the levels of procainamide and N-acetylprocainamide were measured by fluorometry using 0.1 N HCl (32). Two of the normals were fast acetylators as was one of the patients. Peak levels of procainamide in the normals were about 2.5 mcg/ml regardless of acetylator phenotype. However, the levels of N-acetyl procainamide were markedly different. In the fast acetylator, left panel Fig. 3, the N-acetylprocainamide levels rise to over 1 mcg/ml and then slowly declines while in the slow acetylator, right panel, the levels reach only 0.5 mcg/ml.

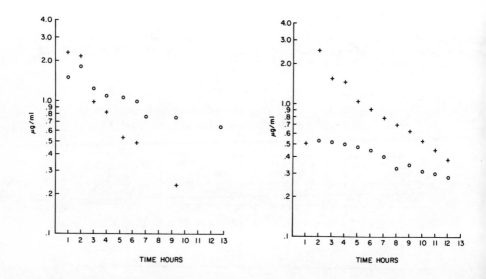

Fig. 3. Log concentration of procainamide (+) and N-acetylprocainamide (o) in serum/time (32). Left panel--subject with normal renal function - rapid INH acetylator. Right panel--subject with normal renal function - slow INH acetylator. Reproduced with permission of publisher.

Figure 4 shows the levels of procainamide and N-acetylprocainamide in an anephric fast acetylator. Because of difficulties with vascular access, sampling was begun 26 hours after the oral dose. At that time the levels of procainamide were 0.5 mcg/ml while those of N-acetylprocainamide were almost

3 mcg/ml. During the next five hours, while on hemodialysis the levels of
both compounds decreased indicating removal by the artificial kidney. After
the completion of dialysis the levels of procainamide continued to decrease
and became undetectable after 37 hours. The levels of N-acetylprocainamide,
in contrast, remained relatively constant and decreased little except during
hemodialysis. N-acetylprocainamide was still measurable in this patient's
serum 123 hours after a single oral dose of procainamide and after three
different hemodialysis treatments. Quite similar results were obtained in
the other two patients.

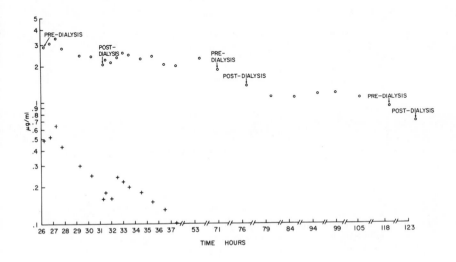

Fig. 4.   Log concentration of procainamide (+) and N-acetyl
          procainamide (o) in serum/time in an anephric rapid
          INH acetylator (32). Reproduced with permission of
          the publisher.

    Although much remains to be determined concerning the therapeutic useful-
ness of N-acetylprocainamide as an antiarrhythmic agent, several studies have
shown that it does have antiarrhythmic activity in a variety of animals and in
man (33,34) Therefore, when treating patients with procainamide, regardless
of the state of renal function, the levels of both compounds must now be taken
into account when assessing the adequacy of therapy. It is conceivable that a
patient may become toxic even though the levels of procainamide are in what is
now considered to be the therapeutic range, 4-10 mcg/ml (5,16) especially if
renal function is impaired.

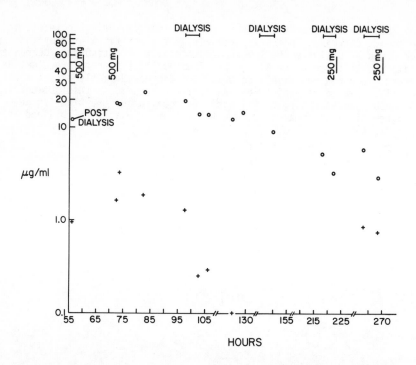

Fig. 5. Log concentration of procainamide (+) and N-acetyl
procainamide (o) in serum/time in an anephric subject
with viral pericarditis. Time is in hours after first
dose.

Figure 5 presents the serum levels of procainamide and N-acetyl
procainamide in a young woman with end stage renal failure, viral pericarditis
and frequent premature ventricular contractions. She had received a total of
1 gram of procainamide HCl prior to the first serum sample which was taken at
the completion of hemodialysis 55 hours after the first dose and 44 hours
after the second dose. At that time the levels of N-acetylprocainamide and
procainamide were 12.1 mcg/ml and 0.9 mcg/ml, respectively. Twelve hours
after an additional 1 gram of procainamide HCl (85 hours, Fig. 5), the serum
level of N-acetylprocainamide was 24 mcg/ml while the level of procainamide
was 1.8 mcg/ml. Thereafter, the levels of N-acetylprocainamide declined very
slowly except when hemodialysis intervened. At 125 hours, when procainamide
was no longer detectable in serum the level of N-acetylprocainamide was 13.5
mcg/ml and decreased to 6 mcg/ml at 215 hours.

If the levels of procainamide alone had been used as a guide to dosing
frequency, it is probable that very high levels of N-acetylprocainamide would
have accumulated. High levels could lead to toxic manifestations in the form

of new arrhythmias and hypotension that might be attributed to the underlying disease state. On the other hand, in the absence of measurable levels of procainamide, if the rhythm returned to normal, further therapy might be withheld, the thought being that the underlying condition has resolved, when in fact the levels of N-acetylprocainamide were therapeutic.

Up to now we have been discussing the effect of the absence of renal function on the elimination of procainamide and the accumulation of N-acetylprocainamide and have not discussed the effect of hemodialysis on the removal of these compounds.

The factors determining the ability of a given artificial kidney to remove a given substance are a) protein binding, b) molecular size, c) volume of distribution (V_d), and d) characteristics of the dialyzer.

Procainamide is about 15% protein bound and N-acetylprocainamide, 11% (32). Both are, therefore, readily diffusible and should be easily dialyzable. The molecular weight, procainamide 219 Daltons and 261 Daltons for N-acetylprocainamide, of both is relatively small, and again of little consequence except that it might be expected on the basis of this one parameter that N-acetylprocainamide would not be as readily removed as would procainamide.

The plasma clearance (CL_T) of any drug is defined by the following relationship (34):

$$CL_T = V_d \times k_e \qquad \text{(Eq. 1)}$$

where:

V_d volume of distribution

k_e elimination rate constant and is equal to $0.693/T_{\frac{1}{2}}$

Therefore, CL_T will vary directly with changes in V_d and inversly with changes in $T_{\frac{1}{2}}$.

The V_d of a drug will have a great influence upon the ability of any dialyzer to enhance the intrinsic plasma clearance. During clinical hemodialysis, if there is no change in the inherent metabolic processes a new CL_T, CL_{TD} is established:

$$CL_{TD} = CL_T + CL_D \qquad \text{(Eq. 2)}$$

where:

CL_D dialyzer clearance in ml/hour

In the past the efficiency of a dialyzer has been measured in terms of clearance, expressed as ml/minute. Although such a representation is acceptable, a more meaningful estimation of the effectiveness of a dialyzer can be obtained if its contribution to overall elimination is expressed as the fractional amount (FR) of a substance removed per unit time:

$$FR = 1 - e^{-kt} \qquad\qquad (Eq.\ 3)$$

where:

$k \quad CL_T/V_d$

$t \quad$ time

During dialysis:

$$FR = 1 - e^{-(CL_{TD}/V_d)t} \qquad\qquad (Eq.\ 4)$$

To illustrate the interaction of V_d on the efficiency of an artificial kidney during clinical hemodialysis let's examine the following situation for a given drug (Fig. 6): Subject weight, 70 kg; $k_e = 0.1$ hr^{-1}; dialysis clearance, 100 ml/min; time on dialysis, 1 hour.

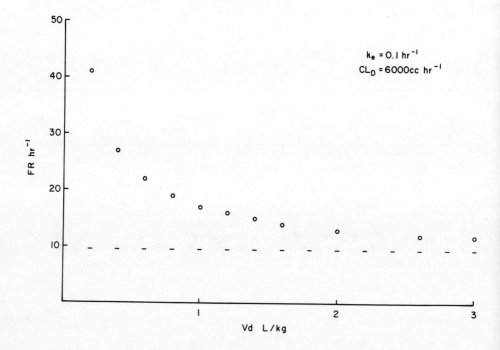

Fig. 6. Effect of increased volume of distribution (V_d) on the fractional amount removed (FR).

In this situation, the V_d is varied from 0.2 to 3.0 L/kg. The horizontal dashed line represents the FR of the inherent metabolic processes which are assumed to remain constant during hemodialysis. The curvilinear line represents the effect of increasing V_d on the total FR. As V_d increases the contribution of the dialyzer to the total FR decreases and asymptotically approaches the inherent FR. Factors that would decrease CL_D, such as protein binding, would diminish the contribution of the dialyzer to the total FR. A more efficient dialyzer would increase the total FR. The most important point to be made is that as V_d increases the contribution of the dialyzer to the total FR will decrease regardless of the clearance in terms of ml/minute. A possible exception to this would be the case of those drugs with very long half lives. In this instance a very modest clearance of 20 ml/minute would greatly increase the overall CL_T.

The relationship that exists between the percent change in CL_T with dialysis and the percent decrease in the $T_{1/2}$ as a result of dialysis is shown in Fig. 7. It is a straight line with a slope of one. Therefore, it is possible to predict the effect of a given artificial kidney on the $T_{1/2}$ of any compound if CL_T and CL_{TD} are known. For such a relationship to be of any clinical usefulness the V_d of drugs commonly used in renal failure must be known.

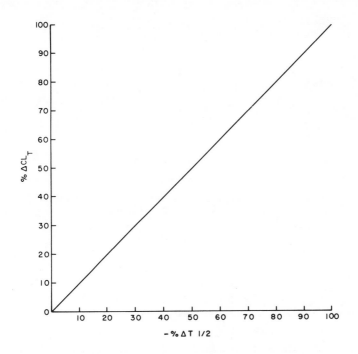

Fig. 7.   Relationship between % change in plasma clearance (CL_T) and % change in half life ($T_{1/2}$).

199

The volume of distribution of procainamide in normal man ranges from 1.76 to 2.6 L/kg (16,31,36) while the V_d of N-acetylprocainamide is about 1.38 L/kg (31). The V_d of neither has been determined in renal failure but ou data after oral dosing suggests that the V_d of procainamide is decreased.

Of all the variables affecting the ability of hemodialysis to remove substances, the only one under direct control of the physician is the dialyzer There is now a wide variety of dialyzers from which to choose (37). This being the case, it should be possible to find that dialyzer that is the most efficient for a given compound.

We have studied the clearance of urea, procainamide, and N-acetyl procainamide in six clinically available artificial kidneys. The characteristics of these kidneys are listed in Table III. Clearance studies were done using a 100 L reservoir of standard dialysate to which urea, procainamide, and N-acetylprocainamide were added. The test solution, at a flow of 200 ml/minute was passed through the blood side of the test kidney. Fresh dialysate at a flow of 400 ml/minute was passed through the dialysate side. Venous pressure was maintained at zero. Clearances were calculated in the usual fashion (38).

Table III. Clearance of Urea, Procainamide, and N-acetylprocainamide by Commonly Used Artificial Kidneys

Dialyzer	Surface Area (M2)	Membrane Thickness (micron)	CLEARANCE (ml/min ± S.E.)		
			Urea	Procainamide	N-acetylprocainamide
Dow Model 5	2.5	30	171.0±3.9	114.6±2.4	89.9±2.3
Dow Model 4	1.3	30	141.9±1.6	79.9±5.0	55.3±2.0
Gambro 17	1.02	17	67.7±2.5	50.8±4.7	33.3±4.7
EX 29	1.4	18	155.1±2.8	81.4±0.8	78.0±1.6
EX 25	1.0	18	137.3±1.3	71.6±1.4	62.6±1.9
EX 23	0.84	18	116.6±3.2	50.4±3.1	50.4±2.7

From Table III it can be seen that there are great individual differences in the ability of the dialyzers to clear not only urea, but also procainamide and N-acetylprocainamide. There appears to be no simple relationship between surface area and clearance. Of all the kidneys studied, the Dow model 5, constructed of regenerated cellulose fibers of 30 micron thickness and having a surface area of 2.5 M^2, had the greatest clearance for all test materials. The second most efficient kidney was the EX-29, with a Cuprophan [R] membrane of 18 micron and a surface area of 1.4 M^2. The least efficient, under the test conditions, was the Gambro 17. Normally this kidney is used in situations where ultrafiltration is desired and may have an enhanced clearance under those conditions.

However Table III does allow the physician to make an objective choice of the dialyzer that will most effectively remove these compounds. On the other hand, Table III can be used to select that dialyzer that is the least efficient for the compounds so that during maintenance hemodialysis a minimum amount of drug is removed.

Table IV. Effect of In Vivo Dialysis Clearances on Half
Life of Procainamide and N-acetylprocainamide

	Procainamide[a]	N-acetylprocainamide[b]
	70 kg man	
V_d (L)	123.2 (1.76 L/kg)	96.6 (1.38 L/kg)
$T\frac{1}{2}$ (hr)	11.6	49.5
k_e (hr^{-1})	0.59	0.014
CL_T (L/hr)	7.27	1.36
CL_D (L/hr)	4.02	2.70
CL_{TD} (L/hr)	11.29	4.06
% Δ CL_T	64%	32%
New $T\frac{1}{2}$ (hr)	7.3	15.6
Observed $T\frac{1}{2}$	5.1	7.6

a   UF II in vivo procainamide clearance   67 ml/min
b   EX 23 in vivo N-acetylprocainamide clearance   45 ml/min

In Table IV the in vivo clearances of procainamide and N-acetyl procainamide and dialyzer effects on the $T\frac{1}{2}$ are presented. The clearance of procainamide was obtained using a UF II coil while those for N-acetyl procainamide were from an EX 23 coil. Data on procainamide clearances using the EX 23 coil in vivo are not presented because the levels of procainamide observed approached the lower limit of sensitivity of the method. For this table the V_d of procainamide (1.76 L/kg) and N-acetylprocainamide (1.38 L/kg) are assumed to be the same as in normals. The $T\frac{1}{2}$ of procainamide (11.6 hours) is the mean $T\frac{1}{2}$ of the 20 subjects with end stage renal failure from our previous study. In these studies a UF II coil had an in vivo clearance of procainamide of 67 ml/min. During dialysis there was a 64% increase in the nondialysis CL_T which should give a predicted $T\frac{1}{2}$ of 7.3 hours. The observed $T\frac{1}{2}$ was 5.1 hours. If, however, the V_d of procainamide in renal failure is less than in normal the calculated $T\frac{1}{2}$ would be in closer agreement with the observed.

For N-acetylprocainamide a $T\frac{1}{2}$ in anephrics has not been experimentally obtained after administration of N-acetylprocainamide alone. However, the $T\frac{1}{2}$ in anephrics can be estimated using the methods described in Chapter 10. In the presence of normal renal function:

$$k_e = k_r + k_{nr} \qquad \text{(Eq. 5)}$$

where:

k_r renal excretion rate constant

k_{nr} nonrenal excretion rate constant

The renal excretion rate constant, k_r, is defined as:

$$k_r = A_u^\infty \cdot k_e/\text{amount of drug absorbed} \qquad \text{(Eq. 6)}$$

where:

A_u^∞ amount of unchanged drug recovered in the urine over 7 half lives

For N-acetylprocainamide A_u^∞ has been found to be 87% (31). In renal failure Eq. 5 reduces to:

$$k_e = k_{nr} \qquad \text{(Eq. 7)}$$

Using Eq. 7 the expected $T\frac{1}{2}$ of N-acetylprocainamide in an anephric patient is 49.5 hours.

Referring back to Table IV with an in vivo dialysis clearance of N-acetylprocainamide of 45 ml/min, CL_{TD} is three times greater than CL_T and the predicted $T\frac{1}{2}$ is 15.6 hours. The observed $T\frac{1}{2}$, 7.6 hours, is one half the predicted value. Using the experimentally obtained $T\frac{1}{2}$ of 7.6 hours, we calculated that the V_d should be 0.7 L/kg. In a personal communication, Dr. Arthur Atkinson, Jr., has noted in a patient taking a large dose of procainamide who required dialytic intervention because of serious toxicity and shock, a V_d for N-acetylprocainamide of 0.7 L/kg. In this case an EX 23 coil was also used.

The important point to be made with respect to the application of dialyzer clearance data is that this data taken alone does not allow the prediction of the end result of dialysis. In Table IV it can be seen that the clearance of N-acetylprocainamide in terms of ml/min is less than the clearance of procainamide. However, the net effect of hemodialysis on the total body burden is much greater.

We strongly feel that data similar to that presented above is needed for all pharmaceuticals. Such dialysis data combined with the pharmacokinetic parameters of V_d, $T\frac{1}{2}$ and protein binding in renal disease will permit a better prediction of the end result of hemodialysis. For toxic overdose in patients with normal renal function the same is true.

In conclusion, it has been shown that in end stage renal failure the $T\frac{1}{2}$ of procainamide is prolonged and N-acetylprocainamide, an active metabolite accumulates and may reach therapeutic levels. The expression of the efficiency of an artificial kidney in terms of its clearance alone has been shown to be of little value. What is important is the contribution of the dialyzer to the overall plasma clearance. To obtain such information the volume of distribution, half life, and protein binding of drugs in renal failure must be known.

References

1. E. G. Lowerie, J. M. Lazarus, C. L. Hampers and J. P. Merrill. Cardio-vascular disease in dialysis patients. New Eng. J. Med. 290:737-738 (1974).
2. A. Lindner, B. Charra, D. J. Sherrard and B. H. Scribner. Accelerated atherosclerosis in prolonged maintenance hemodialysis. New Eng. J. Med. 290:698-701 (1974).
3. B. Lown, A. M. Fahkro, W. B. Hood, Jr. and G. N. Thorn. The coronary care unit: New perspectives and directions. J. Am. Med. Assoc. 199:188-198 (1967).
4. B. N. Chiang, L. V. Periman, L. D. Ostrander and F. H. Epstein. Relationship of premature systoles to coronary heart disease and sudden death in the Tecumseh Epidemiologic Study. Ann. Int. Med. 70:1159-1166 (1969).
5. J. T. Bigger, Jr. and R. H. Heissenbuttel. The use of procainamide and lidocaine in the treatment of cardiac arrhythmias. Prog. Cardiovas. Dis. 11:515-534 (1969).
6. A. L. Bassett and B. F. Hoffman. Antiarrhythmic drugs: Electrophysio-logical actions. Ann. Rev. Pharmacol. 11:143-170 (1971).
7. B. F. Hoffman, M. R. Rosen and A. L. Wit. Electrophysiology and pharma-cology of cardiac arrhythmias. VII. Cardiac effects of quinidine and procainamide.B. Am. Heart J. 90:117-122 (1975).
8. H. J. Conn, Jr. and R. J. Luchi. Some cellular and metabolic consider-ations relating to the action of quinidine as a prototype antiarrhythmic agent. Am. J. Med. 37:685-699 (1964).
9. C. T. Ueda, D. S. Hirschfeld, M. M. Scheinman, M. Rowland, B. J. Williamson and B. S. Dzindzio. Disposition kinetics of quinidine. Clin. Pharmacol. Ther. 19:30-36 (1976).
10. K. M. Kessler, D. T. Lowenthal, H. Warner, T. Gibson, W. Briggs and M. M. Reidenberg. Quinidine elimination during impaired cardiac or renal function. New Eng. J. Med. 290:706-710 (1974).
11. R. Levy, A. Seller, W. J. Mandel and R. Okun. Quinidine pharmacokinetics in anephric and normal subjects. Clin. Res. 24:85A (1976).
12. H. L. Conn, Jr. and R. J. Luchi. Some quantitative aspects of the binding of quinidine and related quinoline compounds by human serum albumin. J. Clin. Invest. 40:509-516 (1961).
13. M. A. Rossi and B. Lown. The use of quinidine in cardioversion. Am. J. Cardiol. 19:234-238 (1967).
14. L. C. Mark, H. J. Kayden, J. M. Steele, J. R. Cooper, I. Berlin, E. A. Rovenstine and B. B. Brodie. Physiological disposition and cardiac effects of procainamide. J. Pharmacol. Exp. Ther. 102:5-15 (1951).
15. H. J. Kayden and B. B. Brodie. Procainamide: A review. Circ. 15:118-126 (1957).
16. J. Koch-Weser. Pharmacokinetics of procainamide in man. Ann. N.Y. Acad. Sci. 179:370-382 (1971).
17. H. S. Weily and E. Genton. Pharmacokinetics of procainamide. Arch. Int. Med. 130:366-369 (1972).
18. T. P. Gibson, D. T. Lowenthal, H. A. Nelson and W. A. Briggs. Elimination of procainamide in end stage renal failure. Clin. Pharmacol. Ther. 17:321-329 (1975).
19. J. Koch-Weser and S. W. Klein. Procainamide dosage schedules, plasma concentrations, and clinical effects. J. Am. Med. Assoc. 215:1451-1460 (1971).

20. J. Dreyfuss, J. T. Bigger, Jr., A. I. Cohen and E. C. Schreiber. Metabolism of procainamide in rhesus monkey and man. Clin. Pharmacol. Ther. 13:366-377 (1972).
21. C. A. Bratton and E. Marshall, Jr. A new coupling component for sulfanilamide determination. J. Biol. Chem. 128:378-382 (1939).
22. E. Matusik and T. P. Gibson. Fluorometric assay for N-acetylprocainamide. Clin. Chem. 21:1889-1902 (1975).
23. S. Whittingham, I. R. Mackay, J. A. Whitworth and G. Sloman. Antinuclear response to procainamide in man and laboratory animals. Am. Heart J. 84:228-234 (1972).
24. R. R. Hope and L. A. Bates. The frequency of procainamide induced systemic lupus erythematosus. Med. J. Aust. 2:298-303 (1972).
25. J. J. Condemi, S. E. Blomgren and J. H. Vaughan. The procainamide induced lupus syndrome. Bull. Rheum. Dis. 20:604-608 (1970).
26. M. M. Reidenberg and J. H. Martin. The acetylator phenotype of patients with systemic lupus erythematosus. Drug.Metab. Dis. 2:71-73 (1974).
27. T. P. Gibson, J. Matusik, E. Matusik, H. A. Nelson, J. Wilkinson and W. A. Briggs. Acetylation of procainamide in man and its relationship to isonicotinic acid hydrazide acetylation phenotype. Clin. Pharmacol. Ther. 17:395-399 (1975).
28. E. Karlsson and L. Molin. Polymorphic acetylation of procainamide in healthy subjects. Acta. Med. Scand. 197:299-302 (1975).
29. M. M. Reidenberg, D. E. Drayer, M. Levy and H. Warner. The polymorphic acetylation of procainamide in man. Clin. Pharmacol. Ther. 19:722-730 (1975).
30. R. L. Galeazzi, L. B. Sheiner, T. Lockwood and L. Z. Benet. The renal elimination of procainamide. Clin. Pharmacol. Ther. 19:55-62 (1976).
31. J. M. Strong, J. S. Dutcher, W. Lee and A. J. Atkinson, Jr. Pharmacokinetics in man of the N-acetylated metabolite of procainamide. J. Pharmacokinet. Biopharm. 3:223-235 (1975).
32. T. P. Gibson, E. Matusik and W. A. Briggs. N-acetylprocainamide levels in patients with end stage renal failure. Clin. Pharmacol. Ther. 19:206-212 (1976).
33. D. E. Drayer, M. M. Reidenberg, R. W. Sevy. N-acetylprocainamide: An active metabolite of procainamide. Proc. Soc. Exp. Biol. Med. 146:358-363 (1974).
34. J. Elson, J. M. Strong, W. Lee and A. J. Atkinson, Jr. Antiarrhythmic potency of N-acetylprocainamide. Clin. Pharmacol. Ther. 17:134-140 (1975).
35. R. E. Cutler, T. G. Christopher, A. W. Forney and A. D. Blair. Modification of drug therapy in chronic dialysis patients. Kid. Int. (Suppl 2): S16-22 (1975).
36. C. Graffner, G. Johnson and J. Sjogren. Pharmacokinetics of procainamide intravenously and orally as conventional and slow release tablets. Clin. Pharmacol. Ther. 17:414-423 (1975).
37. D. N. S. Kerr, N. A. Hoenich, T. H. Frost, C. B. Clayton and D. Jolly. Which dialyzer? Nephron 12:368-392 (1974).
38. A. V. Wolf, D. G. Remp, J. E. Kiley. Artificial kidney function: Kinetics of hemodialysis. J. Clin. Invest. 30:1062-1070 (1951).

Chapter 12

MULTIPLE DOSE PHARMACOKINETICS OF GENTAMICIN IN MAN: EVALUATION

OF THE JELLIFFE NOMOGRAM AND THE ADJUSTMENT OF DOSAGE IN PATIENTS

WITH RENAL IMPAIRMENT

Paul A. Michelson, William A. Miller, John F. Warner,

Leona W. Ayers, and Harold G. Boxenbaum

Gentamicin is a broad-spectrum, bactericidal antibiotic which acts by producing irreversible inhibition of protein synthesis at the bacterial ribosome (1). Its spectrum includes most common Gram-negative and Gram-positive pathogens including E. coli, Kl. aerogenes, Pr. mirabilis, Salmonellae, Shigellae, Neisseriae, H. influenzae, Staph. aureus, and Staph. albus. Most strains of Ps. aeruginosa are also sensitive. The image of gentamicin (1), rightly, is that of a highly potent, moderately toxic drug of immense value in life threatening sepsis.

Many of the clinical aspects of the pharmacokinetics of gentamicin have been reviewed by Schumacher (2-3) and Barza et al (4). One major problem with this drug is that there is a narrow range between effective and toxic serum concentrations. In one recent investigation (5), adequate therapy, based on clinical response, was found to occur when the dose produced peak serum concentrations of 5 µg/ml or more within the first 72 hours of treatment for patients with bacteremia, wound infection, and urinary tract infection. For patients with pneumonia, a level of 8 µg/ml or more was found to be necessary. In adequately treated patients the cure rate was 88%. Although symptomatic ototoxicity was not observed, 18% of the 22 patients exhibited asymptomatic impairment of vestibular function. Other investigators (6-8) have reported that serum gentamicin levels in the range of 12-15 µg/ml may be associated with an increased risk of ototoxicity, especially in the presence of renal failure.

In normal patients (4), the elimination half-life of gentamicin is approximately 2.6 hours. Since the drug is eliminated from the body almost completely by renal excretion, serum level-time profiles are highly dependent on kidney function (2,3). Thus, anephric patients administered gentamicin eliminated the drug from serum with a half-life of 53.4 hours (9).

In view of the low therapeutic index of gentamicin as well as the important role of kidney function on the drug's disposition, several investigators have recommended modified dosage schedules for patients exhibiting varying degrees of renal impairment. Many of these methods have

207

been discussed in the comprehensive reviews of Schumacher (2-3). One particularly interesting and novel method of dosage adjustment has been proposed by Jelliffe (10-14), and a nomogram based on the method is available. This method allows the clinician to pre-select the peak steady-state gentamicin serum level desired, and then to calculate the appropriate intramuscular dosing regimen based on body weight, sex, and renal function.

One purpose of this investigation was to evaluate, and if necessary improve this nomogram in achieving its objectives. In this regard, multiple dose serum gentamicin levels were investigated in 21 hospitalized patients with varying degrees of renal impairment, and these were compared to those levels predicted by the Jelliffe method. It will be demonstrated herein that the Jelliffe method may have predictive value provided a simple adjustment is made. However, as has been reported previously (4, 15), considerable intra and inter-subject variation in observed serum levels may nonetheless be expected.

Theoretical analysis of steady-state serum gentamicin level-time profiles is also presented, and, based on the results, a method of dosage adjustment in renally impaired subjects is recommended.

Theoretical

The Jelliffe nomogram (10-14) for the adjustment of intramuscularly administered gentamicin dosage was developed by employing the linear pharmacokinetic model illustrated in Figure 1. As has been discussed by Wagner and Metzler (16), for the model to have predictive value in a multiple dose situation, it is not necessary for the model to be correct, but rather all that is required is that the equation from the model satisfactorily describe the data. Intramuscularly administered gentamicin is assumed to be completely bioavailable and is absorbed into the body by a first-order process. Drug is then eliminated from the body simultaneously by first-order renal and non-renal processes. It is assumed that a linear relationship exists between the overall elimination rate constant and creatinine clearance, and that the y-intercept of the appropriate plot is the non-renal rate constant (see Figure 1). Following a single intramuscular dose, the time course of serum gentamicin may be described by the following equations (17), where specific values indicated are those utilized by Jelliffe (10-14):

$$C_G = \left(\frac{FD}{V}\right)\left(\frac{k_a}{k_a - k}\right)\left(e^{-kt} - e^{-k_a t}\right) \qquad (Eq. 1)$$

Where: C_G is the serum concentration (μg/ml)

$k = k_r + k_{nr}$

t is time after injection (hours)

F is the bioavailability, taken to be 1.00

D is the dose (μg)

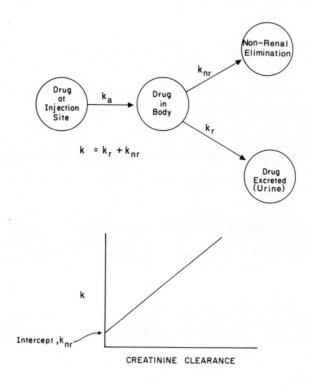

Fig. 1. Absorption and disposition model describing intramuscularly administered gentamicin in man.

V is the volume of distribution, taken to be 15.0% of the body weight in grams, and expressed in ml

k_a is the first-order absorption rate constant, taken to be 2.16 hours[-1]

k_r, k_{nr}, and k are the first-order renal excretion, non-renal elimination, and overall elimination rate constants (hours-1), respectively.

Analogous to the treatment in Chapter 10, the elimination rate constant, k, is calculated from the expression:

$$k = k_{nr} + 0.00324 \, CL_{CR} \tag{Eq.2}$$

Where: CL_{CR} is endogenous creatinine clearance, ml/min

k_{nr} has a value of 0.012 hours[-1]

0.00324 is a constant (slope) having units of min ml[-1] hours-1. The constant 0.00324 multiplied by CL_{CR} is k_r, having units of hours-1.

When a value for creatinine clearance is unavailable, it is calculated from the serum creatinine concentration utilizing the Jadrný equations (18):

For Males:
$$CL_{CR} = \frac{95.94}{C_{CR}^{1.387}} \tag{Eq. 3}$$

For Females:
$$CL_{CR} = \frac{70.31}{C_{CR}^{1.307}} \tag{Eq. 4}$$

where: C_{CR} is serum creatinine concentration, mg/100 ml.

Therefore, from a knowledge of patient body weight, sex, serum creatinine, and dose, a single dose gentamicin serum concentration-time profile can be constructed. The peak level and peak time following single dose administration are given by the following relationships (19):

$$t_{max} = \frac{\ln (k_a/k)}{k_a - k} \tag{Eq. 5}$$

$$C_{G,SD,max} = \left(\frac{FD}{V}\right)\left(\frac{k}{k_a}\right)^{\left(\frac{k}{k_a - k}\right)} \tag{Eq. 6}$$

Where: t_{max} is the time at which a peak serum level is attained following a single dose
$C_{G,SD, max}$ is the peak level following a single dose.

For a 70 kg male subject having a creatinine clearance of 100 ml/min and receiving a single 70 mg intramuscular injection, a peak level of 4.73 µg/ml would be predicted at 1.02 hours.

210

If it is further assumed that serum creatinine, although possibly high, is stable, and that a constant dose of gentamicin is administered at a fixed time interval, the peak steady-state gentamicin serum level may be calculated from the equation developed by Dost (20):

$$C_{G,max} = \left(\frac{FD}{V}\right) \left(\frac{1}{1 - e^{-k\tau}}\right) e^{-\left(\frac{k}{k_a-k}\right)} \ln \left[\frac{k_a\left(1-e^{-k\tau}\right)}{k\left(1-e^{-k_a\tau}\right)}\right] \qquad (Eq.\ 7)$$

Where: C_G, max is the peak steady-state serum gentamicin concentration

τ is the fixed dosage interval

It is now apparent that this latter equation may be easily rearranged to solve for the intramuscularly administered maintenance gentamicin dose required to achieve a pre-selected peak steady-state level. The only experimentally determined parameter required is serum creatinine or creatinine clearance. Moreover, the initial loading dose may be calculated from rearrangement of Equation 6.

The Jelliffe nomogram was constructed based upon the aforementioned equations. Dosage intervals were fixed at 8, 24, or 48 hours for creatinine clearance ranges of 31-125, 11-30, and 0-10 ml/min, respectively. Briefly, the numerical methodology upon which the nomogram is based is as follows:

(a) Serum creatinine, which is assumed to be stable, is used to estimate creatinine clearance using either Equation 3 or 4; alternatively creatinine clearance is directly measured.

(b) The overall elimination rate constant, k, is calculated from Equation 2.

(c) The investigator selects the peak steady-state gentamicin level desired, and the loading dose is calculated from Equation 6; $F = 1$, $V = 15\%$ of body weight, and $k_a = 2.16$ hours^{-1}.

(d) Depending on creatinine clearance, the dosage interval τ has been determined as either 8, 24, or 48 hours, and Equation 7 is next solved to determine the maintenance dose.

One method for evaluating the nomogram would be to experimentally measure peak serum gentamicin levels and determine how well they compare to predicted values. An alternative procedure, which was employed and is reported herein, was to measure serum gentamicin levels at various times during multiple dose therapy, and determine how well these levels were predicted using the aforementioned equations and parameter values. Since it was not always clinically possible to utilize a constant dosing interval, and because serum creatinine values were found to fluctuate to some extent, the principle of superimposition (21-25) was employed with Equation 1 to predict multiple dose gentamicin serum levels. A computer program for a time-shared system was written which calculated serum gentamicin levels by superimposi-

211

tion for a multiple dose regimen. The user entered patient weight, sex, mg doses, times of doses, and serum creatinines at each dose. The principle of superimposition was applied to Equation 1 to calculate multiple dose serum levels at requested times. One interesting feature of the program was that it permitted changes to occur in k, the overall elimination rate constant. When a change in k occurred due to a change in serum creatinine, the residual amount of gentamicin in the body from previous doses were automatically calculated, and gentamicin elimination was thereafter assumed to be governed by the new elimination rate constant.

Using these procedures, it was therefore possible to evaluate the equations and parameters used to construct the Jelliffe nomogram.

Experimental

Patient Selection and Gentamicin Dosing: Twenty-one subjects were recruited from the in-patient population of the Ohio State University Hospitals; intramuscular gentamycin had been prescribed for all patients by their attending physician. Most patients were post-surgical, and many were receiving concomitant medication. No attempt was made to alter the dosing regimen prescribed by the attending physician, and informed written consent was obtained from each volunteer. No attempt was made to control or monitor sites of injection; fortunately, only minor differences in serum concentration-time profiles have been observed following intramuscular administration into thigh or buttock (26). Table I gives the patient characteristics including sex, weight, age, average serum creatinine, creatinine clearance estimated from average serum creatinine, and average hematocrit; also included is information on concomitant medication, gentamicin dosage, average time interval of doses, number of gentamicin doses, and number of blood specimens obtained for analysis of serum gentamicin. Serum creatinine concentrations were generally determined every 1-3 days, depending on the condition of the patient.

All patients received gentamicin sulfate injection, U.S.P. XVIII, each ml containing gentamicin sulfate equivalent to 40 mg gentamicin base (Garamycin (R) injectable, Schering Corporation, Bloomfield, N. J. 07003). Doses reported in Table I are expressed in mg equivalents of gentamicin base.

A special effort was made to obtain blood specimens for serum gentamicin analyses at times at which peak levels would be expected to occur, i.e., approximately one hour after dosing. Additionally, an effort was also made to obtain blood specimens immediately prior to administration of the next dose. Table II gives the frequency at which specimens were obtained in relationship to dosing.

Analytical Methodology: Serum creatinine concentrations were measured by an adaptation of the Jaffe reaction (27) for use on an automatic chemical analyzer (28-29). The microbiological method of Alcid and Seligman (30) was used to determine serum gentamicin concentrations. This procedure employs an antibiotic resistant strain of Staphylococcus epidermidis in an agar well diffusion assay, and has a lower limit of sensitivity of 0.1 µg/ml. The organism was resistant to ampicillin, carbenicillin,

212

Table I

Characteristics of Patients Receiving Intramuscularly Administered, Multiple Dose Gentamycin Therapy

Patient No.	Sex, M or F	Weight, kg	Age, Years	Average Serum Creatinine, mg %	Creatinine Clearance[a], Estimated from Average Serum Creatinine, ml/min
1	M	90.9	48	1.04	120
2	F	59.5	49	0.800	85.3
3	F	57.0	47	0.819	82.7
4	M	67.3	28	1.09	98.1
5	M	66.8	42	1.67	57.1
6	M	88.6	60	1.45	75.9
7	F	66.4	28	1.15	81.9
8	M	80.9	34	0.922	132
9	F	55.9	67	1.55	31.3
10	F	51.8	29	0.900	82.0
11	M	63.2	34	0.900	106
12	M	69.1	42	1.31	75.4
13	M	67.7	65	1.53	51.6
14	F	55.9	42	2.56	16.6
15	M	66.4	64	1.32	59.5
16	F	64.1	43	0.709	115
17	M	73.2	55	1.29	74.0
18	F	68.2	25	0.800	118
19	M	84.5	33	0.767	167
20	M	60.0	54	0.800	98.7
21	F	66.8	51	1.60	46.2

a Calculated from Equations 9-10.

Table I (cont'd)

Characteristics of Patients Receiving Intramuscularly Administered, Multiple Dose Gentamicin Therapy

Patient No	Average Hematocrit, %	Gentamicin Therapy Post Surgery, Yes or No?	Concomitant Anti-bacterials	Gentamicin Doses, mg
1	42.9	Yes	None	80
2	34.9	Yes	None	60
3	33.4	Yes	Clindamycin	80, 60
4	40.3	No	Cephalexin	80
5	33.0	Yes	None	80
6	38.0	Yes	Sulfameth-oxazole Ampicillin	80
7	35.0	Yes	None	80
8	43.2	Yes	Ampicillin	60
9	28.4	?	None	50
10	32.4	Yes	None	60
11	39.8	No	None	60
12	34.0	Yes	None	80
13	42.1	Yes	Ampicillin	80
14	31.6	Yes	None	60
15	34.5	Yes	None	75
16	35.2	Yes	Nitrofuran-toin, Cepha-loridine	60
17	35.2	Yes	None	60
18	33.8	No	Clindamycin	80
19	36.7	Yes	Carbenicillin	80
20	36.5	Yes	Tetracycline	80
21	24.4	No	Clindamycin	60

Table I (cont'd)

Characteristics of Patients Receiving Intramuscularly Administered, Multiple
Dose Gentamicin Therapy

Patient No.	Average Time Interval of Doses, Hours	No. of Gentamycin Doses	No. of Serum Specimens Obtained
1	8.58	20	3
2	8.00	13	2
3	7.93	37	7
4	11.5	16	5
5	7.86	15	5
6	7.90	6	2
7	7.95	19	2
8	7.94	9	2
9	14.2	6	2
10	7.95	6	2
11	7.50	21	8
12	8.13	27	5
13	9.18	8	3
14	12.0	10	3
15	11.9	8	2
16	8.08	11	3
17	8.22	10	2
18	8.19	11	2
19	7.93	6	1
20	7.75	13	3
21	12.3	5	2

Table I. (Cont'd)

Characteristics of Patients Receiving Intramuscularly Administered, Multiple
Dose Gentamicin Therapy

Patient No.	Diagnosis or Surgery	Concomitant Conditions
1	Kidney Stones	Pyelonephritis
2	Commissurotomy	Pneumonia
3	Hysterectomy	Infection
4	Acute Epididymitis	Urinary Tract Infection
5	Ventricular Septal Repair	Pneumonia
6	Prostatectomy	None
7	Hysterectomy	Infection
8	Vesicoctomy	None
9	Urinary Bladder Cancer	Urinary Tract Infection
10	Hysterectomy	Infection
11	Epididymitis	Diabetes
12	Ventricular Septal Repair	Pneumonia
13	Sacral Cyst	None
14	Aortic Valve Replacement	None
15	Prostate Operation	Urinary Tract Infection
16	Severe Low Back Pain	None
17	Mitral Valve Replacement	None
18	Pelvic Inflammatory Disease	None
19	Uretopelvic Junction Obstruction	Urinary Tract Infection
20	Supraglottic Laryngectomy	None
21	Colonic Adrenocarcinoma	Urinary Tract Infection

Table II.   Distribution of Times after Intramuscular Gentamicin Doses
that Bloods were drawn for Serum Gentamicin Determinations.

Time Elapsed from Previous Dose, hours	No. of Serum Samples Analyzed
0-0.25	1
0.51-0.75	1
0.76-1.00	21
1.01-1.25	12
1.26-1.50	4
1.51-1.75	2
1.76-2.00	3
2.01-2.25	1
4.75-5.00	1
5.01-5.25	1
6.26-6.50	1
6.76-7.00	1
7.01-7.25	2
7.26-7.50	5
7.51-7.75	1
8.01-8.25	1
8.26-8.50	1
9.01-9.25	1
11.01-11.25	1
11.26-11.50	2
11.51-11.75	1
11.75-12.00	1

cephalothin, chloramphenicol, tetracycline, kanamycin, streptomycin, colistimethate, sulfisoxazole, lincomycin, and clindamycin. Additional studies (31) have indicated no interference exists in the assay due to the presence in serum of tetracycline HCl (6 µg/ml), sulfamethaxazole (75 µg/ml), cephaloridine (50 µg/ml), cephalexin monohydrate (50 µg/ml), nitrofurantoin (5 µg/ml), and ampicillin (10 µg/ml), alone, or all 6 compounds in combination. Thus, the organism used in this assay was unaffected by all the concomitant antimicrobial agents administered to the patients in this investigation as listed in Table I.

Results and Discussion

Predictions Based Upon the Jelliffe Equations and Parameters: As indicated previously, a computer program was developed which applied the principle of superimposition and determined multiple dose serum gentamicin levels based upon Equations 1-4. The user entered doses, times of administration, and serum creatinines at each dose. Since serum creatinines were not determined as frequently as were the doses administered, values from the most recent determination were used. As indicated previously the program was flexible in the sense that it could handle changes in the elimination rate constant, as indicated by changes in serum creatinine.

Using this program, it was possible to generate theoretical serum gentamicin-time profiles for any dosing regimen. Figure 2 illustrates a theoretical profile for subject 5 based on data from this subject. Also illustrated in this figure are measured serum gentamicin concentrations. The data from the subject typifies the results generally obtained, that is, that theoretical levels substantially over-estimated measured levels. This is illustrated from the data of all patients in Figures 3 and 4. Figure 3 is a plot of measured vs. theoretical gentamicin serum levels. Ordinate values were weighted by the factor 1/y, and a straight line equation was fitted by least-squares linear regression. Application of the appropriate t test (32) indicated that the intercept was not significantly different from zero (p > 0.05), but that the slope was significantly different from 1 (p < 0.05). This finding that the slope differed from 1 indicated a systematic error in the method of calculation of theoretical gentamicin serum levels. This point is better illustrated in Figure 4, which is a plot of percent deviation vs. theoretical gentamicin serum concentration. Percent deviation was determined from the relationship:

$$\text{Percent Deviation} = \frac{\left(\begin{array}{c}\text{Theoretical}\\\text{Serum Level}\end{array}\right) - \left(\begin{array}{c}\text{Measured}\\\text{Serum Level}\end{array}\right)}{1/2\left[\left(\begin{array}{c}\text{Theoretical}\\\text{Serum Level}\end{array}\right) + \left(\begin{array}{c}\text{Measured}\\\text{Serum Level}\end{array}\right)\right]} \times 100 \qquad \text{(Eq. 8)}$$

The straight line equation was fitted to the data by unweighted least squares analysis. Application of the appropriate t test (32) indicated the slope was not significantly different from zero (p > 0.05). Thus it appears that the theoretical method over-estimates the actual gentamicin serum levels by a nearly constant factor. It shall be demonstrated subsequently that this factor is approximately 1.4, i.e., the Jelliffe method predicts

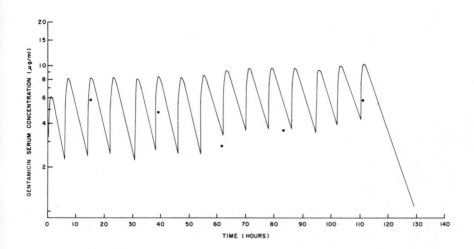

Fig. 2.   Theoretical gentamicin serum level-time profile
          following multiple dose administration to subject
          5 using the intramuscular route. Curves were gener-
          ated using the Jelliffe parameters and equations;
          measured serum levels are also illustrated.

serum levels approximately 1.4 times greater than those actually measured.
Alternatively, it may be stated that the measured multiple dose serum
gentamicin levels are approximately 71% of those predicted. Also, referring
to Figure 4, it is quite interesting to note that at the lower predicted
levels, the percent deviations were greatest.

     Some comment on the calculation of percent deviation seems appropriate.
The equation used produces the same absolute values of percent deviation
when the measured levels differ from the theoretical levels by any factor or
the reciprocal of that factor. For example, consider the case where the
theoretical level is 1.4 µg/ml and there exist measured levels of 2.24 and
0.875 µg/ml, respectively. The former measured level differs from the calculated level by a factor of 0.625, whereas the latter measured level differs
by a factor of 1/0.625. However, the percent deviations are identical,
i.e., 46.2%, except that the signs are opposite. In cther words, an observed
level twice the calculated level produces the same absolute percent deviation
as an observed level half the calculated level. Therefore, in calculating

219

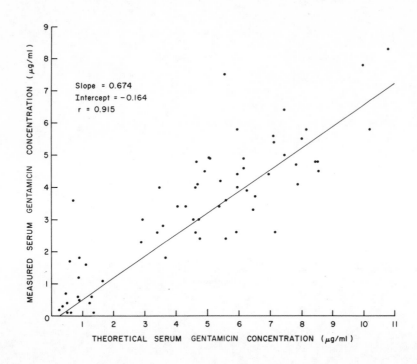

Fig. 3. Relationship between measured serum gentamicin levels and
those obtained theoretically from the Jelliffe parameters
and equations. Ordinate values were weighted by the factor
1/y, and a straight line equation was fitted by least-squares
linear regression.

percent deviations from Equation 8, it was felt that, clinically, observed
values twice the calculated values were just as much in error as observed
levels half the calculated levels.

Adjustment of the Jelliffe Parameters: From observation of Figure 4, it is
readily apparent that a systematic error (or errors) exists somewhere in the
Jelliffe numerical approach. Potential sources of errors considered were
with respect to the values of the absorption rate constant, the slope and
intercept values of the creatinine clearance-elimination rate constant plot,
the bioavailability, and the volume of distribution. Initially, the
absorption rate constant of 2.16 hours^{-1} was critically examined. As indicated previously, using this value with a subject having a creatinine
clearance of 100 ml/min, a peak level at 1.02 hours is calculated from
equation 5 for a subject receiving a single intramuscular dose. This is in
general agreement with many other investigators (33-38), who observed peak
levels approximately one hour after intramuscular injection. The numerical

220

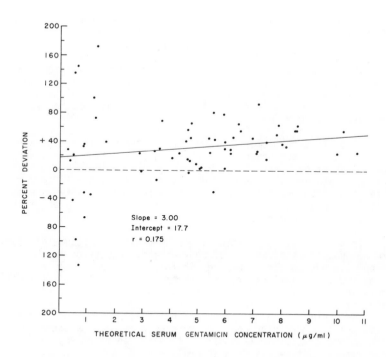

Fig. 4. Relationship between percent deviations and theoretical
serum gentamicin levels calculated from the Jelliffe
parameters and equations. A straight line equation
was fitted by unweighted least-squares linear regression.

values of the slope and intercept of the linear relationship between elimination rate constant and creatinine clearance were also scrutinized (the possibility of a non-linear relationship of these parameters will be discussed shortly). The intercept value of 0.012 hours^{-1}, i.e., k_{nr}, corresponds to an elimination half-life of 57.8 hours in the complete absence of renal function, i.e., a creatinine clearance of zero. Interestingly, Lockwood and Bower (9) reported an average elimination half-life of 53.4 hours in five anephric patients. Therefore, the k_{nr} value appears to be reasonably accurate. Using the value of 0.00324 min ml^{-1} hours^{-1} for the slope, and assuming k_{nr} to be correct, a subject with a creatinine clearance of 100 ml/min would have a calculated elimination rate constant of 0.336 hours^{-1}; this corresponds to an elimination half-life of 2.06 hours, and is in excellent agreement with the mean value of 2.0 hours reported by Lockwood and Bower (9) for 10 subjects with normal kidneys. However, as reviewed by Kaye et al (15), the reported elimination half-lives of gentamicin in patients with normal renal function have varied widely in different studies. Additionally, Kaye et al (15) analyzed sets of data from 5 different groups of investigators, and performed a linear regression analysis of elimination rate constant-creatinine clearance data, only using creatinine clearance data in the range of 30-120 ml/min. The value of the slope was determined as 0.0022 min ml^{-1} hours^{-1}, and the intercept was 0.07 hours^{-1}. These values differ considerably from the slope and intercept values of .00324 min ml^{-1} hours^{-1} and 0.012 hours^{-1}, respectively, used by Jelliffe. Perhaps even more relevant to the discussion is the data of Barza et al (4) who reported that elimination rate constant-creatinine clearance plots were non-linear. These data were acquired from 42 patients, 13 of whom had estimated CL$_{CR}$ values less than 30 ml/min.

The one clear fact that emerges from all the various investigations is that there exist wide intersubject variations in elimination half-lives, and that these variations cannot be explained solely on the basis of differences in creatinine clearances. For example, the data of Barza et al (4) indicate wide differences in elimination half-lives in patients with normal renal function. The wide intersubject variability has been discussed by both Kaye et al (15) and Barza et al (3).

As discussed previously, Equation 1 was used with the volume of distribution term being calculated as 15% of body weight. Any error in this parameter would be systematic in nature, in that all serum levels at all times are inversely proportional to this parameter. Therefore, theoretical multiple dose serum levels could be altered in such a way to increase or decrease them by a constant factor simply by altering the volume of distribution term. Referring again to Figures 3 and 4, it is apparent that there exists a systematic error which could be corrected to a large extent by altering the volume of distribution term. It was determined empirically, by trial and error, that by assuming the volume of distribution to be 21.1% of body weight, the average percent deviation was essentially zero. Using this value of 21.1%, theoretical values of serum gentamicin concentrations were recalculated, and Figure 5 illustrates a plot of measured vs. theoretical serum gentamicin levels. Application of the appropriate t statistic (32) indicated that the slope and intercept did not differ significantly from 1 and zero, respectively (p > 0.05). Figure 6 illustrates a plot of % deviation vs. theoretical serum gentamicin levels, and the t test indicated that both the slope and intercept values did not differ significantly from from zero (p >0.05). Thus it may be concluded that adjustment of the volume of distribution term resulted in a considerable improvement of the Jelliffe method. Schumacher (2,3) has also challenged the 15% figure employed by Jelliffe, and has recommended a 20% value. (Note that the gentamicin simulations presented previously in Chapter 10 Figure 11 utilized the 20% value.)

Nonetheless, in spite of this correction and improvement, there still remains a basic problem. Although Figures 5 and 6 suggest randomness of scatter of the ordinate functions, this is somewhat misleading. This is clarified in Table III, which indicates that the mean % deviation for most patients differs considerably from zero. Therefore, one could expect measured gentamicin serum concentrations to deviate considerably in individual patients from the predicted or theoretical values. In other words, inter-subject variation is considerable, and that the pooling of all data from all subjects tends to mask systematic errors in individual subjects. Additionally, it is also apparent from Table III that inter-subject variation is also considerable.

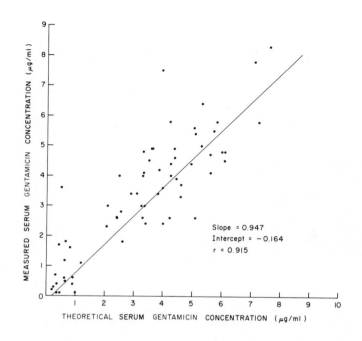

Fig. 5. Relationship between measured serum gentamicin levels
and those obtained theoretically from the Jelliffe parameters
and equations, but by assuming the volume of distribution
to be 21.1% of body weight. Regression was performed as
in Figure 3.

Although it appeared that the best possible fit between theoretical and
measured serum levels was attained by this procedure, it still remained to be
verified whether or not systematic errors could be attributed to measured
physiological parameters. In this respect, the values for % deviations were
correlated with: (a) time after last dose; (b) hematocrit; (c) serum creatinine; (d) age; and (e) weight. The correlation coefficients were, respectively, -0.026, +0.0840, -0.00251, -0.0974, and +0.0619. Once again, application of the appropriate t-test (32) indicated that all the slopes of the
linear least squares regression lines were not significantly different from
zero (p > 0.05). Additionally, visual examination of the data revealed no
apparent correlation between % deviation and sex.

Application of the Siersbaek-Nielsen and Co-Workers Method for Determination
of Endogenous Creatinine Clearance Based Upon Subject Weight, Age, Sex, and
Serum Creatinine: In the previous discussion, serum creatinine levels were
used to calculate endogenous creatinine clearances based upon the Jadrný

223

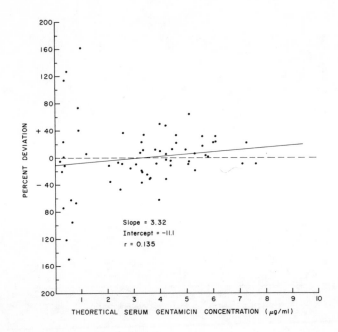

Fig. 6. Relationship between percent deviations and theoretical
serum gentamicin levels calculated from the Jelliffe
parameters and equations, but by assuming the volume of
distribution to be 21.1% of body weight. Regression was
performed as in Figure 4.

equations (18) utilizing data solely on the basis of sex and serum creatinine. More recently, Siersbaek-Nielsen and co-workers (39-42) developed a
series of equations as well as a nomogram to estimate creatinine clearance
based upon serum creatinine, weight, age, and sex. Since the Jadrny method
(18) does not take into account the variables of weight and age, the
Siersbaek-Nielsen method (39-42) was used to calculate creatinine clearances
in an attempt to reduce the intra and inter-subject variability. Estimation
of CL_{CR} is based on the following equation (39-42):

$$CL_{CR} \text{ (ml/min)} = \frac{\text{Urinary Creatinine (mg/kg/min) x 100 x Weight (kg)}}{\text{Serum Creatinine (mg/100 ml)}} \qquad \text{(Eq. 9)}$$

Values of urinary creatinine (mg/kg/min) x 100 are obtained for males and
females in various age groups. These values are independent of the status
of renal function, since at steady-state, rate of creatinine production
equals rate of creatinine excretion, independent of renal function. This

224

Table III. Percent Deviations Between Measured and Theoretical Gentamicin Serum Concentrations using the Jelliffe Method. Volume of Distribution was taken as 21.1% of Body Weight

Subject #	No. of Serum Specimens Obtained	Mean % Deviation	% Deviation Lowest Value	Highest Value
1	3	+14.2	+7.65	+23.6
2	2	-31.5	-63.5	+0.599
3	7	+46.6	+11.9	+127.
4	4	+51.6	-62.0	+163.
5	5	+9.20	-8.86	+22.4
6	2	+40.6	+33.7	+47.5
7	2	-7.34	-18.6	+3.85
8	2	+0.850	-35.6	+37.3
9	2	-36.8	-67.0	-6.58
10	2	+27.6	+22.4	+32.7
11	8	-42.0	-151.	-10.0
12	5	+1.33	-10.3	+11.6
13	3	+41.9	+30.1	+64.6
14	3	-16.3	-30.9	-8.59
15	2	-109.	-122.	-95.4
16	3	-24.6	-46.8	-5.85
17	2	-27.3	-29.8	-24.7
18	2	+26.7	+13.0	+40.4
19	1	-16.5	-16.5	-16.5
20	3	-3.52	-11.3	+5.71
21	2	-17.6	-31.4	-3.82

was verified experimentally (39-42).

The Siersbaek-Nielsen and co-workers method was modified so that it could be accurately used with digital computer methods. Average urinary creatinine excretion rate values were obtained (39-42) for males and females having serum creatinines $\leq$ 1.4 mg/100 ml and being in the age groups of 20-29, 30-39, 40-49, 50-59, 60-69, 70-79, 80-89, and 90-99 years. Average values of urinary creatinine excretion rates, (mg/kg/min) x 100, in males and females, were plotted as a function of the midpoints of the age groups (i.e., 24.5, 34.5, 44.5 years, etc.); the appropriate plots are illustrated in Figure 7. A fourth degree polynomial equation was fitted to the data

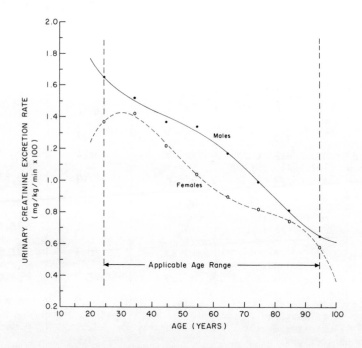

Fig. 7. Urinary creatinine excretion rate as a function of age. A fourth degree polynomial equation was fitted to the two sets of data by unweighted regression analysis.

using unweighted regression analysis (43):

$$y = ax^4 + bx^3 + cx^2 + dx + e \qquad \text{(Eq. 10)}$$

This equation was fitted to the two sets of data, where the y values are

226

urinary creatinine excretion rates, (mg/kg/min) x 100, and the x values are the midpoints of the age groups. The coefficients are given below, and the fitted curves are illustrated in Figure 7:

Coefficient	Males	Females
a	$.12515051 \times 10^{-6}$	$-.29299681 \times 10^{-6}$
b	$-.30493269 \times 10^{-4}$	$.72486697 \times 10^{-4}$
c	$.25532217 \times 10^{-2}$	$-.63411621 \times 10^{-2}$
d	$-.98885908 \times 10^{-1}$	$.21683517$
e	2.94759	-1.09193

Thus by substituting the patient's age in the appropriate polynomial expression, an estimate of urinary creatinine excretion rate, (mg/kg/min) x 100, could be obtained. Equation 9 could then be employed to estimate creatinine clearance from serum creatinine. An important requirement necessary for the correct application of this procedure is that creatinine excretion rate is not dependent upon renal function. Assuming that serum creatinine is stable, and that steady-state conditions exist, and further assuming creatinine does not undergo metabolism, then the rate of creatinine excretion should equal rate of production, independent of renal function. Kampmann et al (39,41) did indeed find that creatinine excretion rates in particular age groups were unaffected by renal impairment.

The aforementioned procedure was employed in the present gentamicin analysis, in an attempt to ascertain whether or not calculation of creatinine clearance as discussed above had any practical advantages over the Jadrný method. Once again, theoretical gentamicin serum levels were calculated as previously described, assuming that volume of distribution was 15% of body weight. As anticipated, theoretical levels here also considerably over-estimated the measured levels. It was empirically determined, by trial and error, that when the volume of distribution was taken to be 20.5% of body weight that the average % deviation was essentially zero. Figure 8 illustrates a plot of measured vs. theoretical serum gentamicin levels, and Figure 9 illustrates a plot of percent deviation vs. theoretical serum gentamicin concentrations. In Figure 9, the appropriate t tests (32) indicate that the slope and intercept values do not differ significantly from zero (p > 0.05), and in Figure 8, the t tests indicate that slope and intercept values do not differ significantly from 1 and zero, respectively (p > 0.05). Therefore, it may be concluded that, overall, within the context of the present discussion, a reasonable fit and randomness of scatter has been achieved by this procedure. Nonetheless, there still exists a great deal of intra and inter-subject variability, and the visual inspection of the appropriate plots indicates that this procedure did not achieve a better fit of measured serum concentrations to the theoretical values than did the previous method employing the Jadrný equations. This result should not in any way be construed as a commentary on the use of the Siersbaek-Nielsen and co-workers method of converting serum creatinine values to creatinine clearance. Indeed, the authors favor and recommend this method. Rather, the only point

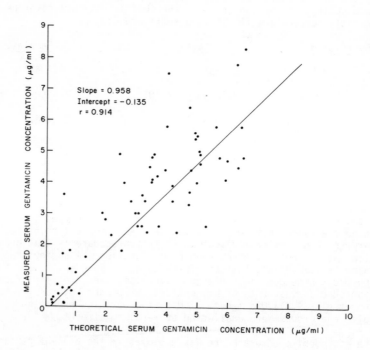

Fig. 8. Relationship between measured serum gentamicin levels and those obtained theoretically using the Jelliffe method but employing the modified Sierbaek-Nielsen and co-workers method for estimation of creatinine clearance. Volume of distribution was taken to be 20.5% of body weight; regression was performed as in Figure 3.

intended here is that this method offers no advantage over the Jadrny method in predicting gentamicin serum levels when used with the Jelliffe equations with the data obtained in this particular experiment only.

Application of the Barza and Co-Workers Method for Determination of Gentamicin Elimination Rate Constants: Barza et al (4) applied multiple linear regression techniques to gentamicin serum data following single doses, and developed linear regression equations to estimate gentamicin elimination half-lives in terms of sex, serum creatinine concentration, and reciprocal of hematocrit. For males, the elimination half-life of gentamicin is obtained by the following equation:

$$t_{1/2} = -3.68 + 0.898\ C_{CR} + \frac{258}{(\%\ \text{hematocrit})} \qquad (Eq.\ 11)$$

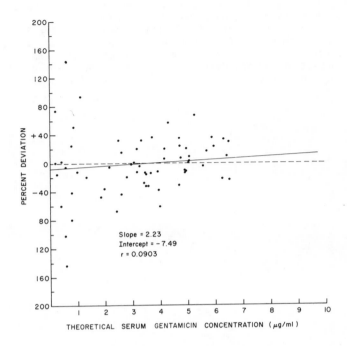

Fig. 9. Relationship between percent deviation and theoretical serum gentamicin levels calculated using the Jelliffe method but employing the modified Siersbaek-Nielsen and co-workers method for estimation of creatinine clearance. Volume of distribution was taken to be 20.5% of body weight; regression was performed as in Figure 4.

For females, the following equation was used:

$$t_{1/2} = -5.02 + 0.898\ C_{CR} + \frac{258}{(\%\ \text{hematocrit})} \qquad (Eq.\ 12)$$

where $t_{1/2} = \ln 2/k$, and

% hematocrit = 100 x hematocrit

Equations 11 and 12 were used with the data from this present investigation to determine elimination rate constants and to calculate theoretical serum gentamicin levels, as previously described. Once again, the absorption rate constant was taken to be 2.16 hours⁻¹. It was empirically determined, by trial and error, that a volume of distribution representing 30.9% of

229

body weight gave an average % deviation of essentially zero. Barza et al (4) estimated volume of distribution to be 32.4% of body weight, which is in close agreement to the value empirically determined here. The 30.9% value was utilized with the data from this investigation, and Figure 10 illustrates a plot of measured vs. theoretical serum gentamicin levels, and Figure 11 illustrates a plot of percent deviation vs. theoretical serum gentamicin concentration. In Figure 11, the appropriate t tests (32) indicate that,

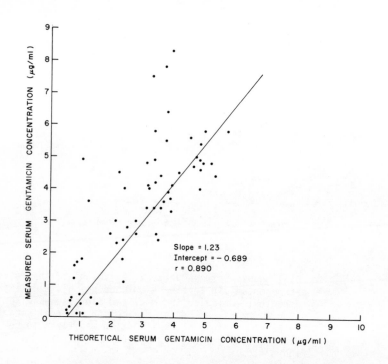

Fig. 10. Relationship between measured serum gentamicin levels and those obtained theoretically using a model with elimination half-lives determined by the method of Barza et al. Volume of distribution was taken to be 30.9% of body weight; regression was performed as in Figure 3.

while the estimate of the intercept does not differ significantly from zero (p > 0.05), the estimate of the slope does differ significantly from zero (p ≤ 0.05). In figure 10, both the slope and intercept values differ significantly from 1 and zero, respectively (p ≤ 0.05). Therefore, it may be concluded that application of Equations 11 and 12 to the data obtained from this present investigation, applied with the constraints of the Jelliffe method, results in a systematic scatter of measured gentamicin serum levels about the theoretical values. As shall be discussed subsequently, this finding should not be construed as indicating any shortcomings or errors in the findings of Barza et al.

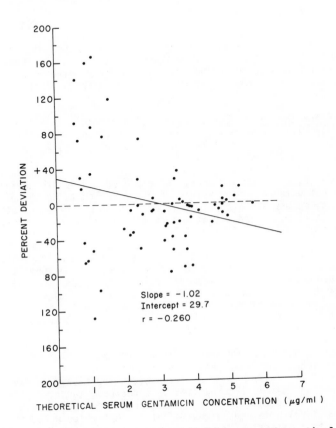

Fig. 11. Relationship between percent deviation and theoretical serum gentamicin levels calculated from a model with elimination half-lives determined by the method of Barza et al. Volume of distribution was taken to be 30.9% of body weight; regression was performed as in Figure 4.

An expected finding arises from the treatment of these data in calculating elimination rate constants by the equations of Jelliffe (10-14) and Barza et al (4). For normal male patients (hematocrit 0.45, serum creatinine 1.0 mg %), the Jelliffe and Barza et al equations predict elimination rate constants of 0.323 and 0.235 hours^{-1}, respectively. The empirically determined values of volume of distribution were 21.1 and 30.9% of body weight, respectively. Total body clearance (CL_T) may be calculated (17) from the equation:

$$CL_T = kV \qquad (Eq. 13)$$

For a 70 kg man, the Jelliffe and Barza et al equations give similar CLT values of 79.5 and 84.7 ml/min, respectively. This is necessary, since the average gentamicin equilibrium serum level, $\bar{C}_G$, is given by (17, 44):

$$\bar{C}_G = \frac{FD}{kV\tau}$$

(Eq. 14)

where τ is a fixed dosing interval. If $\bar{C}_G$ is to remain constant for given values of F, D, and τ, then kV must remain constant. In other words, no matter which method is used to derive equations and parameter values consistent with a single set of multiple dose data, total body clearance will remain relatively constant.

Recommendations for the Intramuscular Dosage of Gentamicin in Patients with Renal Impairment: It is apparent that when a correction is made, the Jelliffe method and nomogram has some degree of predictability. An interesting facet of the Jelliffe method is that it allows the clinician to pre-select a peak steady-state serum gentamicin concentration. As discussed previously, however, a correction should be employed. Since the Jelliffe nomogram was constructed assuming volume of distribution to be 15% of body weight, and because a figure of 21.1% appears to be more consistent with our data, it is recommended that the dose attained with the present nomogram be multiplied by the factor 21.1/15, i.e., 1.4. In other words, if the nomogram is to be used, it is recommended that the dose derived from the nomogram be multiplied by 1.4, and this dose administered to achieve the selected peak steady-state gentamicin serum level. Additionally, as will be discussed shortly, it is recommended that the nomogram of Siersbaek-Nielsen and co-workers (40) be used to determine CL_{CR} and that this latter value be used as an index of renal function. Alternatively, the recently developed equations of Cockcroft and Gault (45) may be employed. These equations will be discussed subsequently.

An alternative approach for the adjustment of dosage regimens of drugs in patients with renal impairment has been discussed by Tozer (46). The essential basis of the method is to either prolong the dosage interval (dose remains unchanged) or, alternatively, to decrease the dose (dosage interval remains unchanged). In either case, the mean steady-state gentamicin serum level attained is equivalent to that which would be when dosing the drug to a patient with normal renal function. In the context of this discussion, normal creatinine clearance will be considered to be 100 ml/min. The appropriate equation for gentamicin may be written as (46):

$$\frac{D(n)}{D(rf)} = \frac{\tau\ (rf)}{\tau\ (n)} = \frac{100}{3.57 + 0.964\ (CL_{CR,rf})}$$

(Eq. 15)

Where: D(n) is the maintenance dose considered adequate for a normal patient when $CL_{CR} \geq 100$ ml/min;

τ(n) is the fixed dosage interval consistent with the dose D(n) to the normal patient;

D(rf) is the reduced maintenance dose to be administered to a patient with

232

renal impairment, using the normal dosage interval τ (n).

τ(rf) is the prolonged fixed dosage interval at which the normal maintenance dose D(n) is to be administered to a patient with renal impairment.

$CL_{CR,rf}$ is the creatinine clearanee (ml/min) in the renally impaired
subject.

This equation was developed assuming 96.4% of an absorbed gentamicin dose
is excreted intact in the urine of a normal patient with CL_{CR} equal to
100 ml/min as derived from the parameters of Equation 2.

In order to compare the gentamicin serum level-time profiles that
might be expected by applying the various methods of dosage adjustment,
simulations were run for a patient having a CL_{CR} either equal to 100 or
13.6 ml/min. For the purpose of this calculation, it was assumed that the
patient had a weight of 70.0 kg, and that the volume of distribution was
equal to 21.1% of body weight. Results are summarized in Table IV and
Figure 12.

Initially Equation 7 was employed with the Jelliffe method to calculate the appropriate I.M. maintenance dose to be administered every 8 hours
to the normal patient so as to achieve a peak steady state serum level of
7.00 µg/ml; the calculated maintenance dosage regimen was 134 mg every
eight hours, and Figure 12 illustrates the steady state serum level-time
profile during one dosage interval (Case I). The Jelliffe method was then
applied to calculate the appropriate maintenance dose to be administered
every 24 hours to a patient with a CL_{CR} of 13.6 ml/min, so as to once
again achieve a peak steady state serum level of 7.00 µg/ml. The calculated dosage regimen was 83.6 mg every 24 hours (Figure 12 - Case II); the
Jelliffe nomogram pre-selects a dosage interval of 24 hours for values of
CL_{CR} between 11-30 ml/min. One obvious disadvantage of this method of
dosage adjustment is that minimum steady-state serum levels are always
above 2 µg/ml; that is, although the maximum steady-state level is identical to Case I, the minimum level is substantially greater. The next
approach taken was that described by Tozer (46) utilizing Equation 15 to
calculate a reduced dose to be administered every eight hours; the calculated regimen was 22.4 mg every eight hours - Case III. Referring to
Figure 12, it is apparent that the minimum and maximum steady-state
levels are markedly different than from Case I, the patient with normal
renal function; additionally it is also apparent that high serum levels
(> 2.7 µg/ml) are constantly maintained at steady-state. Therefore, another
approach tried was to again apply the Tozer equation (Equation 15), but
this time to calculate a prolonged dosage interval, keeping the usual maintenance dose; the calculated regimen was 134 mg every 48 hours - Case IV.
Referring to Figure 12, it is apparent that this approach results in levels
that closely mimic Case I with respect to the minimum, average, and maximum
steady-state serum gentamicin levels. If one is inclined to use this as a
criterion for dosage adjustment, then this represents a satisfactory approach for the adjustment of gentamicin dosage in patients with renal impairment. An added advantage of this method is that it generally utilizes
doses commercially available in ampules, thereby obviating the need to use

Table IV

Intramuscular Dosage of Gentamicin in a Normal Patient (CL_{CR} = 100 ml/min) and in a Patient with Renal Impairment (CL_{CR} = 13.6 ml/min). Values were Calculated for a 70 kg Subject (V = 21.1% of Body Weight) Using the Model in Figure 1 with the Appropriate Parameters.

Case Number	CL_{CR} (ml/min)	Maintenance Dose (mg)	Dosage Interval (hours)	Average Steady-State Serum Concentration (µg/ml)	Maximum Steady-State Serum Concentration (µg/ml)	Minimum Steady-State Serum Concentration (µg/ml)	Method Utilized to Adjust Dosage in Renal Impairment
NORMAL SUBJECT							
I	100	134	8	3.38	7.00	0.784	None
RENALLY IMPAIRED SUBJECT							
II	13.6	83.6	24	4.21	7.00	2.04	Jelliffe
III	13.6	22.4	8	3.38	3.90	2.74	Tozer (hold τ at 8 hours - adjust maintenance dose)
IV	13.6	134	48	3.38	8.85	0.676	Tozer (hold maintenance dose at 134 mg - adjust dosage interval)

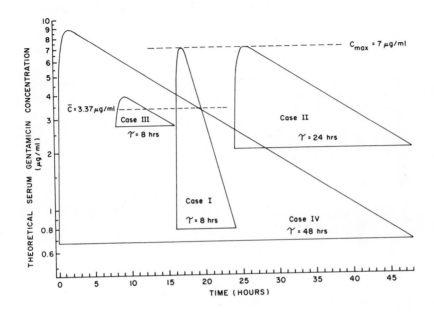

Fig. 12. Theoretical steady-state serum gentamicin level-
time profiles following intramuscular multiple dose
administration. Case I represents a profile of a
subject with normal renal function (CL_{CR} = 100 ml/min),
whereas cases II-IV illustrate profiles attained for
a subject with renal impairment (CL_{CR} = 13.6 ml/min);
these later profiles were obtained by employing
differing methods of dosage adjustment. See Table IV
and text for explanation.

the same ampule to remove small doses on numerous occasions. However, in
patients with severely impaired renal function in which normal doses would
have to be given at intervals exceeding 48 hours, it is recommended that
both the dose and calculated dosing interval be reduced (see recommendations to follow). In all cases, as has been discussed by Tozer (46),
and Welling in Chapter 10, the initial loading dose should not be altered
in the renally impaired patient, i.e., the initial loading dose should be
that loading dose usually administered to a patient with normal renal
function.

One additional factor to be emphasized is that serum creatinine
concentrations below a particular value (e.g., 1-1.2 mg/100 ml) should

not be taken as an index of normal renal function (normal renal function will be considered a CL$_{CR}$ of approximately 100 ml/min). This point is demonstrated in Figure 13, which illustrates plots constructed from the data of Siersbaek-Nielsen and co-workers (39-42). It is readily apparent

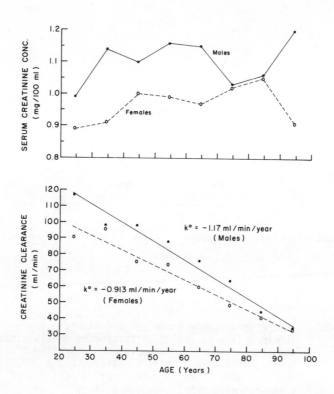

Fig. 13. Relationship between serum creatinine concentrations and renal clearance values. Note the significant reduction of creatinine clearance values with increasing age, without significant changes in serum creatinine levels. Data from references 39-42.

that while serum creatinine levels below 1-1.2 mg/100 ml may be observed in older subjects, these individuals have considerably reduced renal function. The reason for this is quite simple. Serum creatinine at steady-state is equal to creatinine production rate divided by creatinine clearance (creatinine production rate = creatinine excretion rate). In older subjects, both creatinine production rates as well as CL$_{CR}$ are reduced, the net result being little or no change in serum creatinine. From Figure 13, it is interesting to note that CL$_{CR}$ decreases at an approximate zero rate, k^{o}, as a function of age, i.e., beyond the age of 25, CL$_{CR}$ decreases about 1 ml/min/year. Consideration of all the aforementioned factors permits a recommendation to be made for the adjustment of intramuscular gentamicin dosage in patients with renal impairment. The recommendations are:

(a) The initial loading dose should be the loading dose customarily administered to a patient with normal renal function.

(b) The clinician should make a judgment as to the maintenance dose and frequency of administration which he or she would have administered to the patient, assuming normal renal function.

(c) For maintenance therapy, the dose selected above in (b) should be utilized, but the dosing interval should be prolonged according to the equation:

$$\text{Dosing Interval} = \left(\frac{100}{3.57 + 0.964\ CL_{CR}}\right) \left(\begin{array}{l}\text{Frequency of adminis-} \\ \text{tration for patient} \\ \text{with normal renal} \\ \text{function}\end{array}\right)$$

(Eq. 16)

However, if the calculated dosage interval exceeds 48 hours, both the selected normal maintenance dose and calculated dosage interval should be reduced by a constant factor so as to keep the interval under 48 hours. For example if one had calculated a maintenance regimen of 60 mg every 80 hours, a suitable adjustment could be 30 mg every 40 hours.

(d) The value of creatinine clearance for the calculation of the dosing interval, if not measured, should be estimated from serum creatinine, age, weight, and sex using either the nomogram of Siersbaek-Nielsen and co-workers (40) or the equations of Cockcroft and Gault (45).

The method of Cockcroft and Gault (45) for the determination of creatinine clearance is similar to that of Siersbaek-Nielsen and co-workers (39-42). The former investigators plotted creatinine excretion rate vs. age and used linear regression to fit the data; for males the fitted equation was:

Rate of Excretion
(mg/kg/min x 100) $= -0.01389\ \text{Age} + 1.944$ (Eq. 17)

Rearrangement gives the equation:

Rate of Excretion
(mg/kg/min x 100) $= \dfrac{140 - \text{Age}}{72}$ (Eq. 18)

where age is expressed in years in both equations.

Substitution of Equation 18 into Equation 9 gives:

$$CL_{CR} \text{ (ml/min)} = \frac{(140-Age)\,(Wt, kg)}{(72)\,(C_{CR}, mg/100\ ml)}$$
$$(males)$$

To estimate creatinine clearance in females, 85% of the male value is used. This method gives creatinine clearance values similar to those from the nomogram of Siersbaek-Nielsen and co-workers (45).

Intra and Inter-Subject Variability of Gentamicin Serum Levels:
Possible Relationship to the Component Nature of the "Gentamicin Complex": A reading of the recent literature (4, 15) indicates
that there is a strong consensus of opinion that gentamicin serum levels
are generally "unpredictable". In fact, one article (15) is entitled
"The Unpredictability of Serum Concentrations of Gentamicin: Pharmacokinetics of Gentamicin in Patients with Normal and Abnormal Renal Function".
Barza et al (4) have stated that "... the predictability of the $t_{1/2}$ of
gentamicin on the bases of sex, age, body weight, serum creatinine, BUN, and
hematocrit in patients with renal impairment is far from satisfacroty".

One explanation for the observed variability in serum gentamicin levels
could be related to the nature of the chemical composition of the drug.
The drug gentamicin is in fact a mixture of three chemical entities, gentamicin C_1, C_{1a}, and C_2 (47). The United States Food and Drug Administration
permits the complex to contain, by weight, the following ranges of
components:

gentamicin C_1	25-50%
gentamicin C_{1a}	15-40%
gentamicin C_2	20-50%

Separation of the three components is achieved by employing descending
paper chromatography, and the individual substances are eluted into
phosphate buffer. The activities of the components relative to a standard
are subsequently determined using a microbiological agar diffusion assay
employing Staphyloccoccus epidermidis (ATCC 12228). Total gentamicin is
then calculated from the relationship:

$$\begin{aligned}
\text{Total Gentamicin} &= \frac{\text{Assay of } C_1 \text{ Fraction}}{0.786} + \\[2mm]
\text{(By Weight)} & \quad \frac{\text{Assay of } C_{1a} \text{ Fraction}}{0.977} + \\[2mm]
& \quad \frac{\text{Assay of } C_2 \text{ Fraction}}{1.023}
\end{aligned}$$

(Eq. 19)

The factors of 0.786, 0.977, and 1.023 represent the activities of the
fractions relative to the "gentamicin master standard". The relative
percentages of each of the three terms in Equation 19 must conform to the
limits previously given. The product is subsequently formulated in terms of
overall potency, i.e., relative to the working standard. The master

standard (48-49) was used initially to establish and define the microbiological activity of the working standard, and this working standard was
used for all subsequent work. Both the reference standard and working
standard came from the same lot of material, batch GMC 4J-1-4C of gentamicin sulfate supplied by Schering Laboratories, U.S.A. The relative
composition (by weight) of the components in this batch were:

gentamicin C_1	24.7%
gentamicin C_{1a}	38.9%
gentamicin C_2	36.4%

Therefore, it is apparent that when the drug gentamicin is prescribed,
three chemical entities, each having particular pharmacokinetic properties,
are being administered. If substantial differences in the percentage of
the three components existed from batch to batch, manufacturer to manufacturer, country to country, etc., then this could provide some explanation
for the variability of serum gentamicin levels reported in the literature.
Two laboratories (50-51) have reported the results of their determinations
on different batches of gentamicin, and these are summarized in Table V.
It is apparent that considerable differences may exist between batches.

The next logical question relates to potential differences in bio-
pharmaceutic and pharmacokinetic properties of the components. Subcutaneous
administration to mice of the individual components as well as the complex
resulted in very similar serum level-time profiles (52).

However, in another study (53) employing intravenous and intramuscular
administrations of the complex vs. the C_1 component, serum levels resulting
from equivalent doses of the complex were approximately 1.55 fold that of
the C_1 component. Since the curves were virtually parallel, the differences
most probably reflected differences in tissue distribution, i.e., apparent
volumes of distribution. Therefore, it may be concluded that in man differences in pharmacokinetic parameters do exist between the components.

Five additional factors may in part be responsible for the variability
of results seen in the literature. First, one recent investigation (54)
has found that fever is a principle factor associated with lower levels of
gentamicin. Therefore, some variability might be attributable to the fact
that some studies may have employed febrile patients and other non-febrile
patients. Second, the microbiological methods used to determine serum
gentamicin levels actually measure the sum of antimicrobial potency of the
three gentamicin components. It is conceivable that organisms employed
in the numerous laboratories have different relative potencies (i.e.,
minimum inhibitory concentrations) to the individual gentamicin components.
Therefore, a given gentamicin complex standard (standardized in terms of
activity) theoretically would generate different serum level measurements
between laboratories. That is, if different laboratories use different
organisms with different relative potencies, but all use the same gentamicin
complex standard, then different assay results would be expected. Interestingly, in vitro studies (52) of the susceptibilities of various microorgan-
isms to the individual components C_1, C_{1a}, and C_2 have indicated minimum

239

Table V

Determination of the Percentages of Gentamicin Components, By Weight, in Different Batches of Commercial Material (data from references 50,51).

| Lot # | Percent Weight of Compounds | | |
	C_1	C_{1a}	C_2
1	37.0	27.0	36.1
2	34.0	34.3	31.7
3	39.5	25.2	35.3
4	40.7	26.4	32.9
5	29.7	32.8	37.5
6	38.3	20.6	41.1
7	40.7	21.0	38.4
8	25.2	30.2	44.5
9	34.8	25.1	40.1
10	25.3	29.8	44.9
11	27.7	30.7	41.6
12	29.1	30.5	40.5
Fiducial Limits...	25.2-40.7	20.6-34.3	31.7-44.9

inhibitory concentration ratios of 1:1:1, 2.5:1:2.5, 1:1:2.5, 2.5:2.5:1, and 2.67:1:2.67, respectively for the three components. Therefore, this factor could also contribute to the overall variability. The third factor, and perhaps the one of greatest significance, is the finding in Britain (55-57) that only a minority of the laboratories tested (about 20%) could accurately measure gentamicin in serum. In one evaluation, Reeves (57) reported that when 82 individual laboratories used their own routine standards to measure serum gentamicin levels, 20.7% were rated as providing "good" results, 35.4% "poor" results, and 43.9% "highly misleading" results. Moreover, most of the laboratories initially rated as "good" lost their "good" rating when rated a second time. The obvious query arising from these results relates to the reliability of gentamycin serum level measurements used to study gentamicin pharmacokinetics. Fourthly, the point arises as to the criteria selected by investigators to classify individuals as having normal renal function. As has been discussed previously, and is illustrated graphically in Figure 13, serum creatinine per se cannot be used as an index of renal function. Thus, for example, one investigator might have studied an 80 year female and another a 25 year old male; although both subjects could have had a serum creatinine level of 0.9 mg/100 ml, the two could realistically have had a two-fold difference in creatinine clearance values. However, it is conceivable that both subjects may have been classified as "normal", and differences observed between gentamicin half-lives attributed to inter subject variability. Fifthly, it is clear from the studies of Barza et al (4) that differences in hematocrit can influence gentamicin disposition.

Summary

Twenty-one patients exhibiting varying degrees of renal impairment were used to investigate gentamicin serum levels following multiple dose therapy by the intramuscular route. It was demonstrated that the one-compartment disposition model described by Jelliffe with first-order absorption could reasonably predict serum gentamicin levels, provided the volume of distribution was taken to be 21.1% of body weight. This model assumes a linear relationship between elimination rate constants and creatinine clearance.

A theoretical analysis of steady-state serum gentamicin level-time profiles suggested that the best method for dosage adjustment of gentamicin in renally impaired patients is to utilize the normal maintenance dose, but to prolong the dosage interval. In this regard, simple guidelines were set forth to achieve this objective.

The large intra and inter-subject variability observed with gentamicin serum levels was noted, and it was suggested that much of this variability could be attributed to the component nature of the gentamicin complex. That is, the drug gentamicin is actually a complex of three chemical entities, present in U.S. products in the following allowable percentages, by weight:

Gentamicin C_1	25-50%
Gentamicin C_{1a}	15-40%
Gentamicin C_2	20-50%

Acknowledgments

The authors wish to express their appreciation to Schering Corp., Bloomfield, N. J. 07003, for performing the gentamicin assays used for this paper.

This work was supported in part by a Hoffmann-LaRoche Laboratories Hospital Pharmacy Research Grant.

References

1. T. A. McAllister. Gentamicin in clinical practice. Scott. Med. J. 20:97-98 (1975).
2. G. E. Schumacher. Practical pharmacokinetic techniques for drug consultation and evaluation. IV: Gentamicin blood level versus time profiles of various dosage regimens recommended for renal impairment. Am. J. Hosp. Pharm. 32:299-308 (1975).
3. G. E. Schumacher. Pharmacokinetic analysis of gentamicin dosage regimens recommended for renal impairment. J. Clin. Pharmacol. 15:656-665 (1975).
4. M. Barza, R. B. Brown, D. Shen, M. Gibaldi, and L. Weinstein. Predictability of blood levels of gentamicin in man. J. Inf. Dis. 132:165-174 (1975).
5. P. Noone, J. R. Pattison, and D. G. Davies. The effective use of gentamicin in life-threatening sepsis. Postgrad. Med. J. 50 (Suppl. 7):9-16 (1974).
6. W. L. Hewitt. Reflections on the clinical pharmacology of gentamicin. Acta Pathol. Microbiol. Scand., Section B, 81 (Suppl. 241):151-156 (1973).
7. J. Wersall, P. G. Lundquist, and B. Bjorkroth. Ototoxicity of gentamicin. J. Inf. Dis. 119:410-416 (1969).
8. G. G. Jackson and G. Arcieri. Ototoxicity of gentamicin in man: A survey and controlled analysis of clinical experience in the United States. J. Inf. Dis. 124 (Suppl.):S130-S137 (1971).
9. W. R. Lockwood and J. D. Bower. Tobramicin and gentamicin concentrations in the serum of normal and anephric patients. Antimicrob. Agents and Chemother. 3:125-129 (1973).
10. R. W. Jelliffe, R. Knight, J. Buell, R. Kalaba, and R. Rockwell. Computer assistance for gentamicin therapy. Clin. Res. 18:441 (1970).
11. R. W. Jelliffe. Nomograms for kanamicin and gentamicin dosage. Drug Bulletin, County of Los Angeles, Department of Hospitals, Los Angeles County/University of Southern California Medical Center Therapeutic Committee 5 (No. 2):1-2 (1971).
12. R. W. Jelliffe. Nomograms for kanamicin (K) and gentamicin (G) therapy. In Abstracts of the 11th Interscience Conference on Antimicrobial Agents and Chemotherapy, Atlantic City, N. J., 1971, p. 63.
13. R. W. Jelliffe. Nomogram for gentamicin dosage. Copyrighted, University of Southern California, 1971; a plastic wallet-sized copy of this nomogram is available at the University of Southern California Bookstore for $1.00.

14. R. W. Jelliffe. New development in drug dosage regimens. J. Mond. Pharm. 15:53-78 (1972).
15. D. Kaye, M. E. Levison, and E. D. Labovitz. The unpredictability of serum concentrations of gentamicin: Pharmacokinetics of gentamicin in patients with normal and abnormal renal function. J. Inf. Dis. 130:150-154 (1974).
16. J. G. Wagner and C. M. Metzler. Prediction of blood levels after multiple doses from single-dose blood level data: Data generated with two-compartment open model analyzed according to the one-compartment model. J. Pharm. Sci. 58:87-92 (1969).
17. J. G. Wagner. Biopharmaceutics and Relevant Pharmacokinetics, 1st ed., Drug Intelligence Publications, Hamilton, Illinois, 1971, pp. 242, 245, 292.
18. L. Jadrný. Odhad glomerularni filtrace z. kreatininemie. Casopis Lekaru Ceskych. 104:947-949 (1965).
19. S. Glasstone. Textbook of Physical Chemistry, 2nd ed., D. Van Nostrand Co., Inc., Princeton, N. J., 1946, p. 1077.
20. F. H. Dost. Der Blutspiegel, George Thieme, Leipzig, Germany, 1953, p. 253.
21. W. J. Westlake. Problems associated with analysis of pharmacokinetic models. J. Pharm. Sci. 60:882-885 (1971).
22. W. J. Westlake. The design and analysis of comparative blood-level trials. In J. Swarbrick (ed.), Current Concepts in the Pharmaceutical Sciences: Dosage Form Design and Bioavailability, Lea and Febiger, Philadelphia, Pa., 1973, pp. 149-179.
23. C. D. Thron. Linearity and superposition in pharmacokinetics. Pharmacol. Rev. 26:3-31 (1974).
24. J. G. Wagner. Relevant pharmacokinetics of antimicrobial drugs. Med. Clin. N. America 58:479-492 (1974).
25. B. E. Ballard. Teaching biopharmaceutics at the University of California. Am. J. Pharm. Educ. 32:938-957 (1968).
26. D. S. Reeves, M. J. Bywater, R. Wise, and V. B. Whitmarsh. Availability of three antibiotics after intramuscular injection into thigh and buttock. Lancet II:1421-1422 (1974).
27. M. Jaffe. Über den Niederschlag, welchen pikrinsaure in normalen Harn erzeugh, und über eine neue Reaction des Kreatinins. Ztschr. Physiol. Chem. 10:391-400 (1886).
28. A. L. Chasson, H. J. Grady, and M. A. Stanley. Determination of creatinine by means of automatic chemical analysis. Am. J. Clin. Pathol. 35:83-88 (1961)
29. Technicon Instruments Corporation. Simultaneous Creatinine and Uric Acid. Technicon Autoanalyzer Method File N-30 I/II.
30. D. V. Alcid and S. J. Seligman. Simplified assay for gentamicin in the presence of other antibiotics. Antimicrob. Agents and Chemother. 3: 559-561 (1973).
31. E. Oden. Schering Corp., Bloomfield, N. J. 07003, personal communication.
32. W. J. Youden. Statistical Methods for Chemists, John Wiley and Sons, 1951, pp. 47-49.
33. J. Black, B. Calesnick, D. Williams, and M. Weinstein. Pharmacology of gentamicin, a new broad-spectrum antibiotic. Antimicrob. Agents and Chemother., 1963, pp. 138-147.

34. R. L. Jao and G. G. Jackson. Gentamicin sulfate, new antibiotic against gram-negative bacilli. J. Am. Med. Assoc. 189:817-822 (1964).

35. J. H. Darrell and P. M. Waterworth. Dosage of gentamicin for pseudomonas infections. Brit. Med. J. 2:535-537 (1967).

36. J. C. Gingell and P. M. Waterworth. Dose of gentamicin in patients with normal renal function and renal impairment. Brit. Med. J. 2: 19-22 (1968).

37. J. C. Gingell, G. D. Chisholm, J. S. Calnan, and P. M. Waterworth. The dose, distribution, and excretion of gentamicin with special reference to renal failure. J. Inf. Dis. 119:396-401 (1969).

38. R. E. Winters, K. D. Litwack, and W. L. Hewitt. Relation between dose and levels of gentamicin in blood. J. Inf. Dis. 124 (Suppl.):S90-S95 (1971).

39. J. P. Kampmann, K. Siersbaek-Nielsen, M. Kristensen, and J. M. Hansen. Aldersbetingede variationer i urinkreatinin og endogen kreatininclearance. Ugeskr. Laeger. 133:2369-2372 (1971).

40. K. Siersbaek-Nielsen, J. M. Hansen, J. Kampmann, and M. Kristensen. Rapid evaluation of creatinine clearance. Lancet I:1133-1134 (1971).

41. J. Kampmann, K. Siersbaek-Nielsen, M. Kristensen, and J. M. Hansen. Rapid evaluation of creatinine clearance. Acta Med. Scand. 196:517-520 (1974).

42. B. Lumholtz, J. Kampmann, K. Siersbaek-Nielsen, and J. M. Hansen. Dose regimen of kanamicin and gentamicin. Acta Med. Scand. 196:521-524 (1974).

43. W. J. Dixon (ed.). BMD Biomedical Computer Programs, University of California Press, Berkeley, Calif., 1973, pp. 365-372.

44. J. G. Wagner, J. I. Northam, C. D. Alway, and O. S. Carpenter. Blood levels of drug at the equilibrium state after multiple dosing. Nature 207:1301-1302 (1965).

45. D. W. Cockcroft and M. H. Gault. Prediction of creatinine clearance from serum creatinine. Nephron 16:31-41 (1976).

46. T. N. Tozer. Nomogram for modification of dosage regimens in patients with chronic renal function impairment. J. Pharmacokin. Biopharm. 2: 13-28 (1974).

47. Code of Federal Regulations, Title 21, Food and Drugs, Parts 300 to 499, revised as of April 1, 1975, U.S. Govt. Printing Office, Washington, D.C. 20402, 1975, pp. 197-221, 399-404.

48. L. G. Wayland. Antibiotic Chemistry Branch, National Center for Antibiotic Analysis, Bureau of Drugs, Dept. of Health, Education, and Welfare, Public Health Service, Food and Drug Administration, Washington, D.C. 20204, Personal Communication, Jan. 6, 1976.

49. The International Reference Preparation of Gentamicin, World Health Organization, International Laboratory for Biological Standards, National Institute for Medical Research, Mill Hill, London N.W. 7, England, Jan., 1969.

50. N. Kantor and G. Selzer. Chromatographic separation and bioassay of the gentamicin complex. J. Pharm. Sci. 57:2170-2171 (1968).

51. W. L. Wilson, G. Richard, and D. W. Highes. Chemical determination of component ratio and potency of gentamicin complex. J. Pharm. Sci. 62: 282-284 (1973).

52. J. A. Waitz and M. J. Weinstein. Recent microbiological studies with gentamicin. J. Inf. Dis. 119:355-360 (1969).

53. A. Mosegaard, P. G. Welling, and P. O. Madsen. Gentamicin and gentamicin C_1 in the treatment of complicated urinary tract infections: Comparative study of efficacy, tolerance, and pharmacokinetics. Antimicrob. Agents Chemother. 7:328-332 (1975).
54. J. E. Pennington, D. C. Dale, H. Y. Reynolds, and J. D. MacLowry. Gentamicin sulfate pharmacokinetics: Lower levels of gentamicin in blood during fever. J. Inf. Dis. 132:270-275 (1975).
55. D. S. Reeves. Quality control of gentamicin assays. Lancet II:667-668 (1974).
56. D. McGhie, J. G. P. Hutchison, and A. M. Geddes. Serum-gentamicin. Lancet II:1463-1464 (1974).
57. D. S. Reeves. Accuracy of gentamicin assays. Postgrad. Med. J. 50 (Suppl. 7):20-21 (1974).

SUBJECT INDEX

A

Absorption,
  intestinal, 3,33-48,171
  lag times, 46-47
  rates, 46-47
Acetazolamide, 114
Acetaminophen, 79
Acetylator phenotype, 162-163,
  193-195
Acetylprocainamide, 189-203
Acetylsalicylic acid, 62, 107,
  110
Actin, 116
Age, effect on pharmacokinetics,
  1-2,44,60,101,156,159,
  237-238
Albumin, 62-66,79,82,99-118,
  125,128-134,139-141,144-
  145,147-148
Aldosterone, 21,62
Alkaline phosphatase, 65,79
Alpha adrenergic agents, 23
Alprenolol, 62
Aminohippurate, 156
Aminopyrine, 53,66,80,107
Aminosalicylate, 172
Aminosalicylic acid, 109-110
Amobarbital, 54,59,63-64,
  66,82,107
Amoxicillin, 162
Ampicillin, 54,58-60,63-64,
  162,180
Anemia, 27
Anesthetics, 13-14,21,23
Antimalarials, 104
Antineoplastic agents, 104
Antipyrine, 24,53-54,56,66-67,
  78-80, 82-85
Aprindine, 14

Arabinosyl cytosine, 110
Ascites, 82-83
Aspirin, 62,107,110
Atherosclerosis, 189
Availability,
  extent of, 45-46,64-65,69,71
  89,171,208
  food effects, 89
  rate of, 46-47,88
Azo dyes, 140

B

Bacterial infection, 125,132-
  134,207
Benzpyrene, 24
Beriberi, 22
Bilharziasis, 22
Biliary
  obstruction, 79
  secretion, 53
Bilirubin, 62-65,79,104,107,
  114,133-134,137,139,145-
  146
Bishydroxycoumarin, 108
Blood flow, 13-27,138
  dialysis, 180
  hepatic, 15-25,27,61-62,68-
  71,77-85,99
  iliac, 38
  intestinal, 3,33-38,99
  mesenteric, 38
  muscle, 14
  pulmonary, 13-14
  renal, 25,38,156-158
  skin, 99
  splanchnic, 22-23,37
  splenic, 99

247

Blood urea nitrogen, 158,239
Bone fractures, 101
Bromosulfophthalein, See BSP
Bronchitis, 101,103
BSP, 15,79,81,104,108
BUN, 158,239
Burns, 101

C

Calcified tissue, 104
Cancer, 101-102,104
Carbamazepine, 87-94
Carbenicillin, 162-173
Cardiac failure, 33-48
Cardiopulmonary bypass, 125,
130-134
Cefazolin, 159-160,163,168,
171
Cephalexin, 163,168,180
Cephaloridine, 163
Cephalosporin, 132,173
Cephalothin, 163,168
Chloramphenicol, 53-54,107,162,
168
Chlorcyclizine, 105
Chloroquine, 104
Chlorpromazine, 105
Chlorpropamide, 162
Chlortetracycline, 162
Cholesterol, 5-7
Chromic phosphate colloid, 16
Circulatory collapse, 21,23
Cirrhosis, 21-22,54-55,58-60,
62-63,65,77,102,107-109
Clearance,
  biliary, 61
  dialysis, 197-203
  hepatic, 18-20,61-72,77-85
  intrinsic, 16-19,22,24,61-64
  66,69-72,77-79,81,138-139,
  144-149
  renal, 60,65,157,170
  total, 54-71,138-139,143-145,
  148-149,157,171,197-203,231
Clindamycin, 162,173
Clofibrate, 4-5,108
Cloxacillin, 162,168,171
Cocaine, 104
Colistimethate, 162,180
Congestive heart failure, 3
  14,21,33-48,155
Contraceptives, oral, 101

Corticosteroids, 104,115-116
Corticosterone, 115
Cortisol, 15,24,115
Creatinine, serum, 156,158-159,
  164-165,210-214,223-224,
  227-231,236-239,242
Creatinine clearance, 40,156,
  159-160,163,171,174-178,
  193-194,208-213,220-224,
  227-228,232-233,236-239,
  242
Cyclizine, 105
Cyclopropane, 14,23
Cystic fibrosis, 101,103,108-
  110
Cytochrome P-450, 80

D

Dapsone, 107
Desmethylimipramine, 62,107,
  168
Diabetes, 7,134
Dialyzer clearance, 197-203
Diazepam, 14,54,58-59,66-67,
  106-107
Diazoxide, 168
Dicloxacillin, 106,108-109,
  125,127-129,162
Dicoumarol, 53,112,139-140
Digitoxin, 37,107,125-128,162
Digoxin, 26,37,42-43,105,110,
  116-117,162,168,171-172,
  180
Dihydrofolate reductase, 104-
  105
Dimethylbiguanide, 21,24
Diphenylhydantoin, See
  Phenytoin
Disopyramide, 14
Diuretics, 34,44-48
Diurnal variation, 2
DNA, 104
Dopamine, 25
Doxycycline, 162-164,168,173

E

Edema, 33-34,44
Enzyme
  autoinduction, 87,91
  induction, 56,87,91
Ephedrine, 104

Epilepsy, 87-94
Epinephrine, 134
Erythromycin, 2,162,173
Estradiol, 115
Extraction ratio, 15-25,61-71,
  79

F

Fever, 101,240
First pass effect, 19,39,65,
  69,83,171
Flucytosine, 163,180
Flufenamic acid, 110
Fluorescein, 109
Flurothyl, 7
Folate, 104
Food, effects on bioavailability,
  89
Free fatty acids, 4,5,108,113,
  125-134
Furosemide, 44-48

G

Galactose, 79,81
Gamma globulin, 101,109,113
Gastric
  emptying, 39
  polyps, 102
Gastrointestinal
  absorption, 33-48
  blood flow, 33-38
Genetic factors, 56-57
Gentamicin, 163,173-176,178-180,
  207-242
Globulins, 101,109,113,115
Glomerular filtration, 113,156,
  169-170
Glucagon, 21,24
Glutamic oxalacetic transaminase,
  65,79
Glutamic pyruvate transaminase,
  65,79
Guanidinoacetic acid, 128
Guanidinosuccinic acid, 128

H

Haloperidol, 37
Halothane, 23,26
Heart failure, 33-48
Hematocrit, 212,214,223,228-231,

Hematocrit (Cont.)
  239,242
Hemodialysis, 180,189-203
Heparin, 108,130,134
Hepatic
  blood flow, 15-25,27,61-62,
    68-71,77-85
  clearance, 18-20,61-72,77-
    85
  disease, 53-73,77-85,101-
    102,146-147
Hepatitis
  acute toxic, 102
  acute viral, 54-55,57-59,62-
    63,66-68,73,79,102
  chronic active, 54-56,102
  viral, 22,54-55,57
Hexobarbital, 54,59,66-67
Hydralazine, 193
Hydrochlorthiazide, 14,42
Hydrocortisone, 15,24,115
Hypercalcemia, 155
Hyperlipidemia, 3-7
Hyperlipoproteinemia, 108
Hypertension
  portal, 82
  renovascular, 21-22
Hyperthyroidism, 134
Hypoalbuminemia, 63,101-103,
    108,114,128,132-133,144-
    145,147,149,169

I

Imipramine, 20,105
Indocyanine green, 22,24-25,
  66,78-81,83-85
INH, See Isoniazid
Injection sites, effect of
  blood flow, 14
Insulin, 14
Intact hepatocyte hypothesis,
  80
Intact nephron hypothesis, 156
Intestinal
  absorption, 3,33-48,171
  blood flow, 3,33-38,99
Intrinsic clearance, See
  Clearance
Inulin, 25,156,170
Iodohippurate, 156-158
Iothalamate, 156-158
Isoniazid, 53-54,162,172,193

Isoproterenol, 21,24,26,38,62

J

Jaundice, 139-140,145
Jaundice, obstructive, 54-55

K

Kanamycin, 163
Kernicturus, 145

L

Lactic dehydrogenase, 65
LDH, 65
Leucomethylene blue, 2
Lidocaine, 14,16,19,21-24,26,
    39,54-55,58-59,62,65-66,
    79,110,162,189
Ligandin, 104
Lincomycin, 162
Lipoproteins, 5
Liver
    blood flow, See Hepatic
    disease, See Hepatic
    function tests, 65-66
    perfused rat, 15-16,23
Lupus erythematosus, 193
Lymphatic disease, 102

M

Melanin, 104
Meperidine, 15,54,59,62
Metabolic function, 53-73
Methicillin, 162,180
Methylcholanthrene, 24
Methoxyflurane, 23
Methotrexate, 104-105,110
Methylguanidine, 128
Metolazone, 41
Michaelis-Menten
    kinetics, 18,72,171
    parameters, 61
Minocycline, 159-160,162,168,173
Mixed function oxidase enzymes,
    77-78
Morphine, 24,26,62,109
Mucopolysaccharides, 104
Myalgia, 103
Myocardial infarction, 14,22,42,
    101,134,189

Myosin, 116

N

NADPH-cytochrome-ċ-reductase,
    80
Nafcillin, 162
Neoplastic disease, 101
Nephrotic syndrome, 108,143
Neuroses, 103
Niridazole, 22
Nitrates, organic, 62
Nitroanisole, 80
Nitrofurantoin, 159,168,173
Nitrous oxide, 14,24
Norcyclizine, 105
Norepinephrine, 21,23,26
Nortriptyline, 20,62,65

O

Obstructive jaundice, 54,55
Octanoic acid, 108
Oral availability, See
    Availability
Organic nitrates, 62
Ototoxicity, 207
Ouabain, 37
Oxacillin, 162,180
Oxotremorine, 26
Oxyphenbutazone, 15-16,23
Oxytetracycline, 162

P

PAH, 156
Pamaquine, 104
Para-aminohippurate, 156
Para-aminosalicylate, 172
Para-aminosalicylic acid,
    109-110
Paranoia, 103
Pencillin, 125,127-128,133-
    134,162,168,173,175,178-
    180
Pentazocine, 62
Pentobarbital, 24
Perfusion, See Blood flow
Pericarditis, 196
Peritoneal dialysis, 180
Peritonitis, 101
Phenobarbital, 21,24,25,53-56,
    66,94

Phenothiazines, 104
Phenprocoumon, 24
Phenylbutazone, 53-56,105,107-108,
    110,114
Phenylephrine, 5
Phenytoin, 16,18,55,62-63,66-67,
    72,88,94,106-110,112-114,
    125,127-128,130-134,143-145,
    147-148,168
Portavascular shunt, 19,65,73,78,
    81-84
Pneumonia, 101,207
Prednisolone, 115-116
Prednisone, 56,106,116
Pregnancy, 101
Procainamide, 14,26,39,41-42,
    189-203
Propranolol, 15-16,18,21-24,39,
    65,78,82,112,162
  dextro, 78-80,83,85
  levo, 78
Propylene glycol, 88
Prostaglandin E_1, 5
Protamine sulfate, 130,134
Protein binding, 99-118,125-135,
    137-150,155
  albumin, 5,99-118,125,128-134,
    139-141,144-145,147-148
  plasma, 5,61-64,68-71,82
  renal disease, 107-108,114,116-
    117,125-130,134,168-170
  tissue, 64,103-105,116,117
Prothrombin times, 66,79
Psoralins, 104
Psychoses, 103
Pulmonary stenosis, 38

Q

Quinacrine, 104
Quinidine, 3,26,39-41,107-109,
    189-190

R

Red blood cell/plasma ratio, 15
Renal
  age effects, 60,156,159,237-238,
    242
  blood flow, 25,38,156-158
  clearance, 60,65,157,170
  disease, 101,107-108,114,116-117,
    147,155-181,189-203,207-242

Renal (Cont.)
  function, 155-181,189-203,
    207-242
Renovascular hypertension, 21
Rheumatic fever, 101
Rheumatoid arthritis, 110
Ribitol, 36
Rifampicin, 162

S

Salicylic acid, 53,105,108,114,
    125-128,145-146
Scarlet fever, 101
Schizophrenia, 103
Septicemia, 132
Serum lipids, 4-7
SGOT, 65,79
SGPT, 65,79
Shock, 21-23,132,155,203
Shunts
  intrahepatic, 80
  portasystemic, See Porta-
    vascular
Smoking, 101,142
Sodium/potassium ATPase, 104,
    116
Splanchnic blood flow, 22-23,
    37
Steatosis, 102
Streptomycin, 180
Sulfadiazine, 107-108,162
Sulfadimethoxine, 105
Sulfaethidole, 37
Sulfamerazine, 6
Sulfamethazine, 168-169
Sulfamethoxazole, 125-129,162,
    168,171
Sulfisoxazole, 114,172
Sulphafurazole, See Sulfiso-
    xazole
Sulphadimidine, See Sulfa-
    methazine
Systemic lupus erythematosus,
    193

T

Testosterone, 115
Tetracyclines, 2,104-105,162,
    180
Thiopental, 24,107-108,110
Thrombocytopenia, 190

Ticarcillin, 162,173
Tobramycin, 163
Tolbutamide, 53-55,57-59,62-63,
  66-67
Tonsillitis, 101
Transcortin, 104,115-116
Triamterene, 107,109
Tricuspid insufficiency, 38
Triglycerides, 4-5
Trimethoprim, 162,168,171,180
Trimethylpsoralin, 104
Triolein, 34
Tuberculosis, 1
Tubular
  necrosis, 155
  reabsorption, 113,156
  secretion, 113,156,158,169-170

U

Ultrafiltration, dialysis, 201
Urea, 36,128,156,200-201
Urinary tract infection, 132,173,
  207

V

Vancomycin, 163
Viral
  hepatitis, 22,54-55,57
  pericarditis, 196
Volume of distribution
  acetylprocainamide, 200-201, 203
  age, changes with, 60
  amobarbital, 59
  ampicillin, 58-59
  congestive heart failure,
    reduced in, 3,26,41
  cortisol, 115
  dialysis, effects in, 198-199
  diazepam, 58-60
  dicoumerol, 139-140
  digoxin, 116-117,168
  gentamycin, 176,210,222,229-230
  hexobarbital, 59
  hydrocortisone, 115
  lidocaine, 26, 58-59
  liver disease, changes in, 58-59,
    68,82-83
  meperidine, 59
  penicillin G, 179
  phenytoin, 59,114
  prednisolone, 115

Volume of distribution (Cont.)
  procainamide, 26,200-202
  propranolol, 82-83
  protein binding effects, 64
    107,114,168
  quinidine, 3,41
  renal disease, changes in,
    114,116-117,168,200,202-
    203
  tolbutamide, 59
  warfarin, 59

W

Warfarin, 55,59,66-68,73,108,
  112,137-143,145,147

Single Copies: $9.25 prepaid
APhA Member Rate: $6.50 prepaid

APhA-10
760901